Copyright Notice

Title: Fit at Home: Unlocking Your Potential With Home Workouts
Author: Cali Rowell

Published by Cali Rowell through Kindle Direct Publishing
Saint Cloud, Florida, USA
Cover design by Cali Rowell
Interior layout and design by Cali Rowell

Disclaimer: The information provided in this book is for educational and informational purposes only and is not intended as medical advice. It is not a substitute for professional medical advice, diagnosis, or treatment. Always seek the advice of your physician or other qualified health provider with any questions you may have regarding a medical condition or fitness program. The author and publisher of this book are not responsible for any adverse effects or consequences resulting from the use of the information presented herein.

First Edition: March 2024

Dedication

To all those who aspire to lead healthier lives, may this book be a guiding light on your path to wellness. May it empower you to embrace fitness as not just a goal, but a way of life. Together, let us strive for strength, vitality, and well-being, one step, one rep, at a time.

Table of Contents

Copyright Notice..1

Dedication.. 2

Table of Contents..3

Introduction...7

Workout Routines...9

   Routine 1: Full Body.. 10

   Routine 2: Core Focus..11

   Routine 3: Lower Body Burn................................. 13

   Routine 4: Upper Body Blast............................... 14

   Routine 5: Cardio Burst.................................... 16

   Routine 6: Core and Cardio Combo.......................... 17

   Routine 7: Lower Body Burnout............................. 18

   Routine 8: Upper Body Sculpt.............................. 19

   Routine 9: Core Stability................................. 21

   Routine 10: Cardio Blast.................................. 23

   Routine 11: Total Body Strength............................24

   Routine 12: Core and Flexibility Focus.................... 25

   Routine 13: Quick Cardio Burn............................. 27

   Routine 14: Upper Body Pump............................... 28

   Routine 15: Lower Body Blast...............................30

   Routine 16: Core Stability and Balance.................... 32

   Routine 17: Cardio and Strength Circuit................... 34

   Routine 18: Lower Body Sculpt..............................35

   Routine 19: Upper Body Burn............................... 36

   Routine 20: Core and Cardio Fusion........................38

   Routine 21: Stretch and Relaxation........................ 40

   Routine 22: Full Body Cardio Blast........................ 42

Routine 23: Core and Balance Challenge.....................43

Routine 24: Upper Body Pump and Tone.....................44

Routine 25: Lower Body Burn and Stretch....................45

Routine 26: Total Body Tabata.....................................46

Routine 27: Core and Cardio Quickie......................... 47

Routine 28: Lower Body HIIT......................................48

Routine 29: Upper Body EMOM..................................49

Routine 30: Core and Stretch Finisher........................51

Alternative Workout Equipment.................................53

Alternatives to Dumbbells....................................... 54

Alternatives to Exercise Balls...................................58

Alternative to Resistance Bands................................ 61

Detailed Guide with Modifications and Extensions....... 64

Arm Circles...65

Arm Raises...69

Bicep Curls...73

Bicep Curls to Shoulder Press.................................. 77

Bicycle Crunches... 81

Bird Dogs.. 86

Boat Pose...91

Boxing Punches... 95

Burpees... 100

Butt Kicks.. 104

Calf Raises... 108

Cat-Cow Stretch... 113

Chair Dips..117

Child's Pose... 121

Dead Bug... 125

Fast Feet.. 129

Flutter Kicks.. 133

Flyes...137

Fold Forward.. 142

Glute Bridges.. 146

High Knees..150

Jump Rope..154

Jumping Jacks.. 158

Leg Raises.. 162

Lunges.. 166

Mountain Climber.. 171

Oblique Crunches... 175

Plank.. 179

Pushup... 186

Rows.. 190

Russian Twists... 194

Seated Spinal Twist..198

Seated Toe Touches...203

Shoulder Presses...207

Side Leg Raises... 211

Single Leg Balance.. 215

Single Leg Romanian Deadlifts.........................219

Skater Jumps... 223

Speed Skaters...227

Squats... 231

Standing Quad Stretch.....................................236

Standing Side Bends..240

Supermans...244

Tricep Dips.. 248

Tricep Kickbacks..252

V-ups..256
Wall Sits...260

Introduction

In the hustle and bustle of modern life, finding time for fitness can often feel like an uphill battle. From packed schedules to long commutes, the barriers to achieving our fitness goals can seem insurmountable. Yet, amidst this chaos, there exists a powerful solution that is closer than we realize – the home workout.

Welcome to "Fit at Home: Unlocking Your Potential with Home Workouts." In this book, we embark on a journey to transform the way you approach fitness, empowering you to harness the convenience and flexibility of home-based exercise to achieve remarkable results.

Gone are the days of crowded gyms and expensive memberships. Instead, we embrace the freedom and accessibility of home workouts, demonstrating that you have everything you need to build strength, improve flexibility, and enhance cardiovascular health right within the comfort of your own home.

Whether you're a seasoned fitness enthusiast looking to shake up your routine or a busy professional seeking a practical solution to incorporate exercise into your daily life, this book is your comprehensive guide to unlocking the full potential of home workouts.

From quick 5-minute routines designed for the busiest of days to full-body strength training sessions and targeted flexibility exercises, "Fit at Home" offers a diverse array of workouts to suit every need, preference, and fitness level. With step-by-step instructions and optional modifications and extensions for each move, you'll discover how to maximize your workout efficiency, minimize distractions, and achieve meaningful results in the comfort of your own space.

So, are you ready to embark on this transformative journey? Let "Fit at Home" be your guide as you embark on a path to a fitter, healthier, and happier you – one workout at a time.

Workout Routines

Start each routine with a quick warm-up and finish with stretches to prevent injury. These 5-minute workouts can be done alone or combined for a longer session, based on your schedule and fitness level. Mix and match the routines for longer sessions or alternate them weekly to target different muscle groups. Focus on good form and technique for best results.

These short workouts target various muscles and are easy to fit into your day. Modify exercises as needed for your fitness level and any injuries. They provide a variety of exercises for a quick and effective workout at home. Pay attention to your body and adjust exercises if necessary.

These quick workouts are perfect for busy schedules.

Routine 1: Full Body

Perform each exercise for 1 minute. Detailed instruction and modification can be found at the back of the book.

1. Jumping Jacks

   Start with 1 minute of jumping jacks to get your heart rate up and warm up your entire body.

2. Bodyweight Squats

   Perform bodyweight squats for 1 minute, focusing on keeping your back straight and your knees behind your toes.

3. Push-ups

   Do as many push-ups as you can in 1 minute, maintaining proper form throughout.

4. Plank

   Hold a plank position for 1 minute, engaging your core muscles and keeping your body in a straight line.

5. High Knees

   Finish with 1 minute of high knees, lifting your knees as high as possible while jogging in place.

Routine 2: Core Focus

Perform each exercise for 1 minute. Detailed instruction and modification can be found at the back of the book.

1. Russian Twists

   Sit on the floor with your knees bent and feet lifted. Twist your torso from side to side, touching the floor beside you with each twist.

2. Bicycle Crunches

   Lie on your back, lift your shoulders off the ground, and bring your knees towards your chest. Alternate touching your elbows to the opposite knee.

3. Plank with Shoulder Taps

   Get into a plank position and tap your left shoulder with your right hand, then tap your right shoulder with your left hand. Alternate tapping for 1 minute.

4. Leg Raises

   Lie on your back with your legs straight. Lift your legs towards the ceiling, then slowly lower them back down without touching the floor.

5. Mountain Climbers

Get into a plank position and alternate bringing your knees towards your chest as if you were climbing a mountain.

Routine 3: Lower Body Burn

Perform each exercise for 1 minute. Detailed instruction and modification can be found at the back of the book.

1. Lunges

   Step forward with your right foot and lower your body until your right thigh is parallel to the ground. Alternate legs for 1 minute.

2. Wall Sit

   Find a wall and lower yourself into a seated position with your back against the wall. Hold for 1 minute.

3. Calf Raises

   Stand with your feet hip-width apart and rise up onto your toes, then lower back down. Repeat for 1 minute.

4. Side Leg Raises

   (1 minute each side) - Stand tall and lift your left leg out to the side, then lower it back down. Repeat on the right side for 1 minute each.

5. Squat Pulses

   Lower into a squat position and pulse up and down slightly without coming all the way up. Hold for 1 minute.

Routine 4: Upper Body Blast

Perform each exercise for 1 minute. Detailed instruction and modification can be found at the back of the book.

1. Arm Circles

   (30 seconds each direction) - Stand with your arms extended straight out to the sides and make small circles forward, then backward.

2. Tricep Dips

   Sit on the edge of a sturdy chair or bench with your hands gripping the edge. Lower your body towards the ground by bending your elbows, then push back up.

3. Supermans

   Lie face down on the floor with your arms extended in front of you. Lift your arms, chest, and legs off the ground, then lower back down.

4. Reverse Flyes

   Stand with a slight bend in your knees and hinge forward at the hips. Hold a light weight in each hand and lift your arms out to the sides, squeezing your shoulder blades together.

5. Arm Raises

Hold a weight in each hand and lift your arms straight out in front of you, then lower back down.

Routine 5: Cardio Burst

Perform each exercise for 1 minute. Detailed instruction and modification can be found at the back of the book.

1. Jump Rope or Jumping Jacks

    Start with 1 minute of either jumping rope or jumping jacks to get your heart rate up.

2. Burpees

    Perform as many burpees as you can in 1 minute, starting in a standing position, dropping into a plank, doing a push-up, and then jumping back up.

3. High Knees

    Jog in place, lifting your knees as high as possible for 1 minute.

4. Skater Jumps

    Jump from side to side, landing on one foot and swinging the other behind you, alternating sides for 1 minute.

5. Boxing Punches

    Stand with your feet shoulder-width apart and punch forward with alternating arms, engaging your core muscles.

Routine 6: Core and Cardio Combo

Perform each exercise for 1 minute. Detailed instruction and modification can be found at the back of the book.

1. Mountain Climbers

   Start in a plank position and alternate bringing your knees towards your chest as quickly as possible.

2. Plank Jacks

   Begin in a plank position and jump your legs out wide, then back together, while maintaining a strong core.

3. Flutter Kicks

   Lie on your back with your hands under your glutes. Lift your legs slightly off the ground and kick them up and down in a fluttering motion.

4. Russian Twists with Reach

   Sit on the floor, lean back slightly, and twist your torso from side to side while reaching your hands towards the floor on each side.

5. High Knees with Twist

   Jog in place while lifting your knees high, and twist your torso to touch each knee with the opposite hand.

Routine 7: Lower Body Burnout

Perform each exercise for 1 minute. Detailed instruction and modification can be found at the back of the book.

1. Squat Jumps

    Perform squats, but as you come up, explode into a jump, landing softly back into the squat position.

2. Reverse Lunges

    (1 minute each leg) - Step back with your right leg into a reverse lunge, then return to standing and repeat on the left leg.

3. Calf Raises with Pulse

    Stand on the edge of a step or platform with your heels hanging off. Rise up onto your toes, then lower your heels slightly and pulse up and down.

4. Sumo Squats

    Stand with your feet wider than hip-width apart and toes turned out. Lower into a squat position, keeping your knees in line with your toes.

5. Side Lunge with Knee Drive

    (1 minute each leg) - Step out to the side with your right leg into a side lunge, then drive your right knee up towards your chest. Repeat on the left side.

Routine 8: Upper Body Sculpt

Perform each exercise for 1 minute. Detailed instruction and modification can be found at the back of the book.

1. Push-up Variations

Perform a variety of push-up variations such as standard, wide grip, narrow grip, or incline push-ups for 1 minute.

2. Chair Dips

Sit on the edge of a sturdy chair or bench and place your hands on the edge beside you. Lower your body down by bending your elbows, then push back up.

3. Arm Circles with Weights

Hold a light weight in each hand and make small circles forward for 30 seconds, then reverse the direction for another 30 seconds.

4. Bicep Curls

Hold weights in each hand with your palms facing up. Curl the weights towards your shoulders, then lower them back down with control.

5. Tricep Kickbacks

Hold weights in each hand and hinge forward at the hips. Extend your arms straight back, squeezing your triceps, then return to the starting position.

Routine 9: Core Stability

Perform each exercise for 1 minute. Detailed instruction and modification can be found at the back of the book.

1. Plank with Leg Lifts

    Get into a plank position and lift one leg off the ground, then switch legs, alternating for 1 minute.

2. Side Plank

    Lie on your side with your elbow directly under your shoulder and lift your hips off the ground, holding a side plank position for 30 seconds on each side.

3. Dead Bug

    Lie on your back with your arms extended towards the ceiling and your knees bent at a 90-degree angle. Slowly lower one arm and the opposite leg towards the ground, then return to the starting position and switch sides.

4. Plank with Hip Dips

    Get into a forearm plank position and slowly rotate your hips from side to side, dipping towards the ground without letting your hips touch.

5. V-ups

Lie on your back with your arms extended overhead and your legs straight. Lift your legs and upper body at the same time, reaching your hands towards your feet, then lower back down.

Routine 10: Cardio Blast

Perform each exercise for 1 minute. Detailed instruction and modification can be found at the back of the book.

1. Jumping Lunges

   Start in a lunge position and jump up, switching your legs mid-air to land in a lunge with the opposite leg forward.

2. High Intensity Interval Training (HIIT)

   Perform 20 seconds of high-intensity exercise (such as sprinting in place or high knees) followed by 10 seconds of rest. Repeat for 1 minute.

3. Butt Kicks

   Jog in place while kicking your heels up towards your glutes, focusing on speed and intensity.

4. Squat Jacks

   Start in a squat position, then jump up and land with your feet together before immediately jumping back into a squat.

5. Fast Feet

   Stand with your feet hip-width apart and rapidly tap your feet on the ground as quickly as possible.

Routine 11: Total Body Strength

Perform each exercise for 1 minute. Detailed instruction and modification can be found at the back of the book.

1. Bodyweight Squats

    Perform squats by lowering your body as if sitting back into a chair, then returning to standing position.

2. Push-ups

    Get into a plank position and lower your body by bending your elbows, then push back up.

3. Plank with Alternating Arm Reach

    Start in a plank position, then lift one arm off the ground and reach it straight out in front of you. Alternate arms.

4. Glute Bridges

    Lie on your back with your knees bent and feet flat on the floor. Lift your hips towards the ceiling, squeezing your glutes at the top.

5. Dumbbell Rows

    Hold a dumbbell in each hand and hinge forward at the hips. Pull the weights towards your chest, squeezing your shoulder blades together, then lower them back down.

Routine 12: Core and Flexibility Focus

Perform each exercise for 1 minute. Detailed instruction and modification can be found at the back of the book.

1. Standing Side Bends

   Stand with your feet hip-width apart and arms extended overhead. Lean to one side, keeping your core engaged, then return to center and lean to the other side.

2. Seated Toe Touches

   Sit on the floor with your legs extended in front of you. Reach your arms towards your toes, keeping your back straight.

3. Cat-Cow Stretch

   Get on your hands and knees. Arch your back up towards the ceiling (cat pose), then drop your belly towards the floor and lift your head and tailbone (cow pose).

4. Russian Twists with Leg Extension

   Sit on the floor with your knees bent and feet lifted off the ground. Twist your torso from side to side while extending one leg out straight.

5. Child's Pose

Sit back on your heels with your knees spread apart and arms extended in front of you, resting your forehead on the ground.

Routine 13: Quick Cardio Burn

Perform each exercise for 1 minute. Detailed instruction and modification can be found at the back of the book.

1. Jumping Jacks

    Perform traditional jumping jacks, jumping your feet out wide while raising your arms overhead, then returning to the starting position.

2. Burpees

    Start standing, then squat down, kick your feet back into a plank position, do a push-up, jump your feet back to your hands, and jump up explosively.

3. High Knees

    Jog in place while lifting your knees as high as possible, engaging your core and pumping your arms.

4. Speed Skaters

    Jump from side to side, landing on one foot while extending the other leg behind you and reaching the opposite hand towards the foot.

5. Boxing Punches

    Stand with your feet shoulder-width apart and throw quick punches forward, alternating arms while engaging your core.

Routine 14: Upper Body Pump

Perform each exercise for 1 minute. Detailed instruction and modification can be found at the back of the book.

1. Arm Circles

    Stand with your arms extended out to the sides and make small circles with your arms, first forward, then backward.

2. Diamond Push-ups

    Get into a push-up position with your hands close together under your chest. Lower your body towards the ground, keeping your elbows close to your body.

3. Shoulder Presses with Dumbbells

    Hold a dumbbell in each hand at shoulder height, palms facing forward. Press the weights overhead, fully extending your arms, then lower them back down.

4. Reverse Flyes with Dumbbells

    Bend forward at the hips with a slight bend in your knees, holding a dumbbell in each hand with palms facing each other. Lift the weights out to the sides, squeezing your shoulder blades together.

5. Tricep Dips on Chair

Sit on the edge of a sturdy chair or bench with your hands gripping the edge. Slide your glutes off the chair and lower your body towards the ground by bending your elbows, then push back up.

Routine 15: Lower Body Blast

Perform each exercise for 1 minute. Detailed instruction and modification can be found at the back of the book.

1. Alternating Reverse Lunges

    Step back with your right foot into a lunge, then return to standing and repeat on the left side.

2. Sumo Squats with Calf Raise

    Stand with your feet wider than shoulder-width apart and toes turned out. Lower into a sumo squat, then push through your heels to rise up onto your toes.

3. Single-Leg Romanian Deadlifts

    (1 minute each leg) - Stand on one leg with a slight bend in the knee. Hinge forward at the hips while extending the opposite leg behind you, keeping your back straight. Return to standing and repeat on the other side.

4. Wall Sit with Leg Lifts

    Sit against a wall with your knees bent at a 90-degree angle. Lift one leg straight out in front of you, then switch legs.

5. Squat Pulses

Lower into a squat position and pulse up and down slightly, keeping the tension in your quads and glutes.

Routine 16: Core Stability and Balance

Perform each exercise for 1 minute. Detailed instruction and modification can be found at the back of the book.

1. Bird Dogs

   Start on your hands and knees. Extend your right arm forward and your left leg back, keeping your hips square and core engaged. Return to the starting position and repeat on the other side.

2. Plank with Knee to Elbow

   Get into a plank position and bring your right knee towards your right elbow, then return to plank position. Repeat on the left side.

3. Single-Leg Balance

   (1 minute each leg) - Stand on one leg and lift the other leg off the ground, holding for 30 seconds, then switch legs.

4. Dead Bug with Ball Squeeze

   Lie on your back with a small ball between your knees and elbows. Extend your opposite arm and leg away from each other, then return to the starting position and switch sides.

5. Side Plank with Leg Lift

(1 minute each side) - Get into a side plank position
and lift your top leg up towards the ceiling, then lower
it back down. Repeat on the other side.

Routine 17: Cardio and Strength Circuit

Perform each exercise for 1 minute. Detailed instruction and modification can be found at the back of the book.

1. Jump Squats

    Perform squats, then jump explosively as you come up.
2. Push-up to Side Plank

    Start in a push-up position, perform a push-up, then rotate into a side plank on your right hand. Return to push-up position and repeat on the left side.
3. Mountain Climbers

    Perform mountain climbers, bringing your knees towards your chest as quickly as possible.
4. Reverse Lunges with Front Kick

    (1 minute each leg) - Step back into a reverse lunge, then as you return to standing, kick your right leg straight out in front of you. Repeat on the other side.
5. Plank Jacks

    Start in a plank position and jump your feet out wide, then back together.

Routine 18: Lower Body Sculpt

Perform each exercise for 1 minute. Detailed instruction and modification can be found at the back of the book.

1. Squat to Calf Raise

     Perform squats, then rise up onto your toes into a calf raise at the top.

2. Lateral Lunges

     Step out to the side with your right leg into a lateral lunge, then return to center and repeat on the left side.

3. Glute Bridge Marches

     Lift your hips into a glute bridge position, then march your feet up and down, engaging your glutes and hamstrings.

4. Curtsy Lunges

     (1 minute each leg) - Step your right leg behind your left leg and lower into a curtsy lunge, then return to standing and repeat on the other side.

5. Single-Leg Squats

     (1 minute each leg) - Stand on your right leg with your left leg lifted off the ground. Lower into a squat, then return to standing. Repeat on the other side.

Routine 19: Upper Body Burn

Perform each exercise for 1 minute. Detailed instruction and modification can be found at the back of the book.

1. Wide Grip Push-ups

    Perform push-ups with your hands placed wider than shoulder-width apart.

2. Bent-over Rows with Dumbbells

    Hinge forward at the hips and hold a dumbbell in each hand. Row the weights towards your chest, squeezing your shoulder blades together.

3. Tricep Push-ups

    Start in a plank position with your hands close together under your chest. Lower your body by bending your elbows, keeping them close to your body.

4. Bicep Curl to Shoulder Press

    Hold dumbbells in each hand with palms facing forward. Curl the weights towards your shoulders, then press them overhead.

5. Superman Pulses

Lie face down on the floor with your arms extended overhead. Lift your arms, chest, and legs off the ground, then pulse up and down slightly.

Routine 20: Core and Cardio Fusion

Perform each exercise for 1 minute. Detailed instruction and modification can be found at the back of the book.

1. Plank with Shoulder Taps and Leg Lifts

    Get into a plank position and alternate tapping your shoulders with your hands, while also lifting one leg off the ground at a time.

2. Bicycle Crunches

    Lie on your back with your knees bent and hands behind your head. Alternate bringing your right elbow towards your left knee, then switch sides.

3. Jump Rope

    Mimic jumping rope, hopping on the balls of your feet and swinging your arms in a circular motion.

4. Standing Oblique Crunches

    (1 minute each side) - Stand with your feet hip-width apart and hands behind your head. Lift your right knee towards your right elbow, engaging your obliques. Repeat on the other side.

5. Mountain Climber Twist

Perform mountain climbers, but as you bring your knees towards your chest, twist your torso to the right and left alternately.

Routine 21: Stretch and Relaxation

Perform each exercise for 1 minute. Detailed instruction and modification can be found at the back of the book.

1. Cat-Cow Stretch

   Get on your hands and knees. Arch your back up towards the ceiling (cat pose), then drop your belly towards the floor and lift your head and tailbone (cow pose).

2. Forward Fold

   Stand with your feet hip-width apart and hinge forward at the hips, reaching your hands towards the ground or your feet.

3. Seated Spinal Twist

   (1 minute each side) - Sit on the floor with your legs extended in front of you. Cross your right foot over your left thigh, then twist your torso to the right, placing your left elbow on the outside of your right knee.

4. Child's Pose

   Sit back on your heels with your knees spread apart and arms extended in front of you, resting your forehead on the ground.

5. Standing Quad Stretch

(1 minute each side) - Stand on your right leg and grab your left ankle with your left hand, pulling your heel towards your glutes. Hold for 30 seconds, then switch sides.

Routine 22: Full Body Cardio Blast

Perform each exercise for 1 minute. Detailed instruction and modification can be found at the back of the book.

1. Jumping Jacks

    Perform traditional jumping jacks, ensuring to land softly with each jump.

2. High Knees

    Jog in place while bringing your knees up towards your chest as high as you can, maintaining a brisk pace.

3. Burpees

    Start standing, then squat down, kick your feet back into a plank position, do a push-up, jump your feet back to your hands, and explosively jump up.

4. Mountain Climbers

    Get into a plank position and quickly alternate bringing your knees towards your chest, mimicking a climbing motion.

Routine 23: Core and Balance Challenge

Perform each exercise for 1 minute. Detailed instruction and modification can be found at the back of the book.

1. Plank with Arm and Leg Lift

    Start in a plank position and lift your right arm and left leg simultaneously, then switch sides.

2. Boat Pose

    Sit on the floor with your knees bent and feet flat on the ground. Lean back slightly and lift your feet off the ground, balancing on your sit bones.

3. Side Plank with Rotation

    (1 minute each side) - Get into a side plank position and rotate your torso towards the floor, reaching your bottom hand under your body and then up towards the ceiling. Repeat on the other side.

4. Standing Single-Leg Balance

    (1 minute each leg) - Stand on one leg and lift the opposite knee towards your chest, finding your balance before switching legs.

Routine 24: Upper Body Pump and Tone

Perform each exercise for 1 minute. Detailed instruction and modification can be found at the back of the book.

1. Push-ups with Shoulder Taps

    Perform a push-up, then when returning to the plank position, touch your right hand to your left shoulder, then left hand to right shoulder.

2. Bent-Over Reverse Flyes

    Hold a dumbbell in each hand and hinge forward at the hips. Lift the weights out to the sides, squeezing your shoulder blades together.

3. Tricep Dips with Leg Extension

    Perform tricep dips on a chair or bench, and as you straighten your arms, lift one leg off the ground, then switch legs.

4. Plank Up-Downs

    Start in a plank position on your forearms, then push up onto your hands, one arm at a time, then return to the forearm plank, switching which arm you push up with first each time.

Routine 25: Lower Body Burn and Stretch

Perform each exercise for 1 minute. Detailed instruction and modification can be found at the back of the book.

1. Walking Lunges

    Take a step forward with your right foot and lower into a lunge, then push off your right foot to step forward into a lunge with your left foot.

2. Wall Sit with Leg Lifts

    Sit against a wall with your knees bent at a 90-degree angle. Lift your right foot off the ground, then return it to the wall and switch legs.

3. Standing Calf Raises

    Stand with your feet hip-width apart and rise up onto your toes, then lower back down.

4. Forward Fold with Quad Stretch

    Stand with your feet hip-width apart and hinge forward at the hips, reaching your hands towards the ground. Bend your right knee and grab your right foot with your right hand, pulling it towards your glutes, then switch sides.

Routine 26: Total Body Tabata

Perform each exercise for 20 seconds, followed by a 10-second rest. Repeat the circuit twice for a total of 5 minutes.

1. Squat Jumps

    Perform squats, then explode into a jump as you rise up.

2. Push-ups

    Get into a plank position and lower your body by bending your elbows, then push back up.

3. Mountain Climbers

    Start in a plank position and quickly alternate bringing your knees towards your chest.

4. Russian Twists

    Sit on the floor with your knees bent and twist your torso from side to side, touching the floor beside you with each twist.

5. Burpees

    Begin standing, then squat down, kick your feet back into a plank position, perform a push-up, jump your feet back to your hands, and jump up explosively.

Routine 27: Core and Cardio Quickie

Perform each exercise for 45 seconds, with a 15-second rest between exercises. Repeat the circuit twice for a total of 5 minutes.

1. High Plank with Shoulder Taps

    Get into a plank position and alternate tapping your shoulders with your hands.

2. Flutter Kicks

    Lie on your back with your legs extended and lift them slightly off the ground. Alternate kicking your legs up and down in a fluttering motion.

3. Jumping Jacks

    Perform traditional jumping jacks, jumping your feet out wide while raising your arms overhead, then returning to the starting position.

4. Plank Jacks

    Start in a plank position and jump your feet out wide, then back together.

5. Russian Twists

    Sit on the floor with your knees bent and twist your torso from side to side, touching the floor beside you with each twist.

Routine 28: Lower Body HIIT

Perform each exercise for 40 seconds, followed by a 20-second rest. Repeat the circuit twice for a total of 5 minutes.

1. Squat Jumps

Perform squats, then explode into a jump as you rise up.

2. Reverse Lunges

Step back with your right foot into a lunge, then return to standing and repeat on the left side.

3. Sumo Squats

Stand with your feet wider than shoulder-width apart and toes turned out. Lower into a sumo squat, then push through your heels to rise back up.

4. Lateral Lunges

Step out to the side with your right leg into a lateral lunge, then return to center and repeat on the left side.

5. Jumping Lunges

Perform lunges, but jump into the air and switch legs mid-air to land in a lunge with the opposite leg forward.

Routine 29: Upper Body EMOM

Perform each exercise at the top of every minute for 1 minute, then rest for the remainder of the minute. Repeat the circuit for 5 minutes.

1. Push-ups

    Perform as many push-ups as you can in 1 minute.

2. Bicep Curls with Dumbbells

    Hold dumbbells in each hand with palms facing forward. Curl the weights towards your shoulders, then lower them back down with control.

3. Tricep Dips

    Sit on the edge of a sturdy chair or bench with your hands gripping the edge. Lower your body towards the ground by bending your elbows, then push back up.

4. Shoulder Presses with Dumbbells

    Hold dumbbells in each hand at shoulder height, palms facing forward. Press the weights overhead, fully extending your arms, then lower them back down.

5. Plank Hold

Get into a plank position and hold for as long as you can, aiming for the full minute.

Routine 30: Core and Stretch Finisher

Perform each exercise for 1 minute with a focus on controlled movements and proper form.

1. Dead Bug

    Lie on your back with your arms extended towards the ceiling and your knees bent at a 90-degree angle. Slowly lower one arm and the opposite leg towards the ground, then return to the starting position and switch sides.

2. Seated Forward Fold

    Sit on the floor with your legs extended in front of you and hinge forward at the hips, reaching your hands towards your feet.

3. Cat-Cow Stretch

    Get on your hands and knees. Arch your back up towards the ceiling (cat pose), then drop your belly towards the floor and lift your head and tailbone (cow pose).

4. Side Plank with Rotation

    Get into a side plank position and rotate your torso towards the floor, reaching your bottom hand under

your body and then up towards the ceiling. Repeat on
the other side.

5. Child's Pose

Sit back on your heels with your knees spread apart
and arms extended in front of you, resting your
forehead on the ground.

Alternative Workout Equipment

In the pursuit of fitness and strength, one need not always rely on specialized gym equipment. Household items possess untapped potential as substitutes for conventional workout equipment, offering innovative solutions to maintain fitness goals without the need for specialized gear. With a touch of creativity and resourcefulness, various household items can be repurposed to serve as effective substitutes for traditional workout equipment.

From utilizing water bottles or canned goods as makeshift weights for strength training to repurposing towels or bedsheets for resistance bands, resourcefulness transforms everyday items into effective exercise tools. Even furniture like chairs or countertops can serve as platforms for elevated push-ups or step-ups, while stability and balance can be enhanced using pillows, cushions, or yoga blocks.

By embracing creativity and adaptability, one can seamlessly integrate household items into their workout routines, turning any space into a versatile home gym.

Alternatives to Dumbbells

Some workouts may discuss using weights. When dumbbells aren't available, there are plenty of household items that can be used as substitutes for resistance training. Here are some common household items that can serve as makeshift dumbbells:

1. **Water Bottles or Gallon Jugs:**
   - Fill empty water bottles or gallon jugs with water, sand, or rocks to adjust the weight. These can be used for exercises like bicep curls, shoulder presses, and lateral raises.

2. **Canned Goods or Food Items:**
   - Cans of soup, beans, or other food items with handles can be used as lightweight dumbbells. They're suitable for exercises such as tricep extensions, lateral raises, and overhead presses.

3. **Books or Textbooks:**
   - Stack books or textbooks of varying sizes and weights together to create makeshift dumbbells. Hold them by the spine or covers to perform exercises like bicep curls, overhead presses, and chest presses.

4. **Backpack or Bag with Heavy Items:**
   - Fill a backpack or sturdy bag with heavy items such as books, water bottles, or canned goods. Adjust the weight by adding or removing items as needed. Use the backpack for exercises like squats, lunges, and rows.

5. **Laundry Detergent Bottles or Liquid Containers:**
   - Empty laundry detergent bottles or liquid containers can be filled with water or sand to create makeshift dumbbells. Hold them by the handle to perform exercises like bicep curls, lateral raises, and tricep extensions.

6. **Paint Cans or Home Improvement Supplies:**
   - Large paint cans or containers filled with sand, gravel, or other heavy materials can be used as improvised dumbbells for strength training exercises such as squats, lunges, and overhead presses.

7. **Tote Bags or Grocery Bags:**
   - Fill tote bags or sturdy grocery bags with heavy items like books, canned goods, or bottles to create makeshift dumbbells. Hold the bags by the handles for exercises such as bicep curls, shoulder presses, and lateral raises.

8. **Resistance Bands with Handles:**
   - Resistance bands with handles can simulate many dumbbell exercises and provide adjustable resistance. Anchor the band under your feet or around a sturdy object and perform exercises like bicep curls, shoulder presses, and rows.

9. **Large Water Jugs or Milk Jugs:**
   - Large water jugs or milk jugs filled with water or sand can serve as heavy dumbbells for strength training exercises like squats, lunges, and overhead presses.

10. **Children's Toys or Play Equipment:**
   - Children's toys such as building blocks, stuffed animals, or toy balls can be used as lightweight dumbbells for resistance training exercises. Hold them in your hands to perform exercises like lateral raises, front raises, and bicep curls.

These household items offer versatile alternatives to traditional dumbbells and can be easily adapted to suit your fitness needs and preferences. Just be sure to choose items that are comfortable to hold and provide appropriate

resistance for your strength training routine.

Alternatives to Exercise Balls

When an exercise ball is not available, there are several household items that can serve as substitutes for certain exercises or provide similar benefits. Here are some alternatives:

1. **Chair or Stability Cushion:**
   - A sturdy chair with a backrest can be used for seated exercises that target core stability and balance. Alternatively, a stability cushion or cushioned seat pad can provide an unstable surface similar to an exercise ball, engaging core muscles while sitting.

2. **Pillow or Cushion:**
   - A firm pillow or cushion placed on the floor can be used for exercises that involve lying or kneeling on the ball, such as back extensions or abdominal curls. It provides support while still engaging stabilizing muscles.

3. **Yoga Block or Foam Roller:**
   - A yoga block or foam roller can be used as a substitute for an exercise ball in certain exercises. For example, placing your hands or feet on a yoga block during plank

exercises adds instability and engages core muscles
similarly to using an exercise ball.

4. **Basketball or Soccer Ball:**
   - A basketball or soccer ball can be inflated to a suitable
size and used for exercises that involve rolling or balancing
on the ball. While not as large as an exercise ball, these
balls still provide an unstable surface for core strengthening
exercises.

5. **Large Inflatable Balloon:**
   - A large inflatable balloon, such as a beach ball or yoga
ball, can serve as a makeshift exercise ball for some
exercises. While not as durable or stable as a proper
exercise ball, it can still be used for seated exercises or
balance training.

6. **Rolled-Up Towel or Blanket:**
   - Rolling up a towel or blanket and placing it under the
lower back during exercises like bridges or pelvic tilts can
provide support and stability similar to using an exercise ball.
It also helps maintain proper spinal alignment.

7. **BOSU Balance Trainer:**

- A BOSU (Both Sides Up) balance trainer is a half-dome stability ball with a flat platform on one side. It can be used as an alternative to an exercise ball for balance training exercises, core workouts, and strength training.

8. **Step Stool or Low Platform:**
   - A step stool or low platform can be used for exercises that involve stepping onto or off of the ball, such as step-ups or single-leg balance exercises. It provides a stable surface while still challenging balance and stability.

While these alternatives may not fully replicate the versatility and functionality of an exercise ball, they can still provide effective ways to engage core muscles, improve balance, and add variety to your workout routine. Experiment with different household items to find substitutes that work best for your fitness goals and preferences.

Alternative to Resistance Bands

When resistance bands are not available, there are several household items that can be used as substitutes for resistance training exercises. Here are some alternatives:

1. **Towels or Bed Sheets:**
   - Towels or bed sheets can be used to create makeshift resistance bands by pulling or pushing against the fabric. For example, you can wrap a towel around your feet or hands and use it to perform exercises like bicep curls, rows, or chest presses.

2. **Pantyhose or Tights:**
   - Pantyhose or tights can be stretched to create resistance for various exercises. For example, you can tie knots in the legs of the pantyhose to create handles and use them for exercises like leg lifts, lateral leg raises, or arm curls.

3. **Elastic Bands or Hair Ties:**
   - Elastic bands or hair ties can be used as makeshift resistance bands for exercises that require light to moderate resistance. You can loop them around your hands or feet to

perform exercises like lateral raises, overhead presses, or squats.

4. **Tubing or PVC Pipe:**
   - Tubing or PVC pipe can be used as a substitute for resistance bands by creating loops or handles at each end. You can use the tubing or pipe to perform exercises like bicep curls, tricep extensions, or chest flies.

5. **Rope or Clothesline:**
   - Rope or clothesline can be used to create resistance for pulling exercises such as rows or lat pulldowns. You can anchor one end of the rope to a sturdy object and pull the other end towards you to perform the exercise.

6. **Water Bottles or Gallon Jugs:**
   - Water bottles or gallon jugs filled with water or sand can be used as makeshift resistance weights for exercises like bicep curls, lateral raises, or overhead presses. You can hold them in your hands or loop a towel around them for added grip.

7. **Heavy Books or Textbooks:**

- Heavy books or textbooks can be used as resistance for exercises like chest presses, shoulder presses, or overhead tricep extensions. Hold the books in your hands or press them against your chest or shoulders to create resistance.

8. **Backpack or Bag with Heavy Items:**
   - Fill a backpack or sturdy bag with heavy items such as books, water bottles, or canned goods to create resistance for exercises like squats, lunges, or rows. Wear the backpack or hold the bag while performing the exercises.

While these household items may not provide the same level of resistance or versatility as traditional resistance bands, they can still be effective for strength training exercises when used creatively. Experiment with different items to find substitutes that work best for your fitness goals and preferences.

Detailed Guide with Modifications and Extensions

Arm Circles

Arm circles are a simple yet effective exercise for warming up the shoulders, improving shoulder mobility, and activating the muscles of the arms and upper back. Here are the instructions for performing arm circles, along with modification options and extension exercises:

1. **Starting Position:**
   - Stand tall with your feet shoulder-width apart and your arms extended straight out to the sides at shoulder height.
   - Keep your palms facing down towards the ground and engage your core muscles to maintain stability.

2. **Circular Motion:**
   - Begin by making small circular motions with your arms, moving them forward in a clockwise direction.
   - Gradually increase the size of the circles, making them larger as your shoulders begin to warm up and loosen.
   - Continue circling your arms for the desired number of repetitions or time, aiming for smooth and controlled movements.

3. **Reverse Direction:**

- After completing the desired number of forward arm
circles, switch to circling your arms in a counterclockwise
direction.
   - Start with small circles and gradually increase the size as
your shoulders loosen up.
   - Maintain a steady and controlled pace throughout the
movement, focusing on engaging the muscles of your
shoulders and upper back.

4. **Breathing:**
   - Inhale as you circle your arms forward, drawing air into
your lungs and expanding your chest.
   - Exhale as you circle your arms backward, releasing the
breath and engaging your core muscles for stability.

Modification Options:

1. **Reduced Range of Motion:**
   - If you have shoulder issues or limited mobility, you can
perform smaller arm circles with a reduced range of motion.
   - Start with small circles and gradually increase the size as
your shoulders warm up and become more flexible.

2. **Bent Elbows:**

- If straightening your arms is uncomfortable, you can perform arm circles with slightly bent elbows.
- This modification reduces strain on the shoulder joints while still engaging the muscles of the arms and upper back.

Extension Exercises:

1. **Arm Circles with Resistance Bands:**
   - Hold a resistance band in both hands with your arms extended straight out to the sides at shoulder height.
   - Perform arm circles while holding onto the resistance band, maintaining tension throughout the movement.
   - This adds resistance to the exercise, challenging the muscles of the shoulders and upper back even more.

2. **Dynamic Arm Circles:**
   - Perform arm circles while incorporating dynamic movements, such as stepping forward or backward, lunging, or squatting.
   - This adds a functional component to the exercise, challenging your balance and coordination while engaging multiple muscle groups simultaneously.

3. **Weighted Arm Circles:**

- Hold a light dumbbell or kettlebell in each hand while performing arm circles.
    - The added weight increases the resistance, providing a greater challenge for the muscles of the arms and shoulders.

Arm Raises

Arm raises are a versatile exercise that targets the muscles of the shoulders, upper back, and arms. Here are the instructions for performing arm raises, along with modification options and extension exercises:

1. **Starting Position:**
   - Stand tall with your feet hip-width apart and your arms relaxed at your sides.
   - Engage your core muscles to maintain stability and keep your shoulders relaxed and down away from your ears.

2. **Front Arm Raises:**
   - Begin by lifting both arms straight out in front of you, keeping them parallel to the ground.
   - Keep your elbows slightly bent and your palms facing downwards throughout the movement.
   - Lift your arms until they are shoulder-height or slightly higher, then pause briefly at the top.

3. **Side Arm Raises:**
   - Lower your arms back down to your sides, then lift them out to the sides until they are parallel to the ground.

- Keep your palms facing downwards and your elbows slightly bent throughout the movement.
   - Lift your arms until they are shoulder-height or slightly higher, then pause briefly at the top.

4. **Lowering Phase:**
   - Slowly lower your arms back down to the starting position, resisting gravity to control the descent.
   - Maintain a controlled and steady movement throughout the lowering phase.

5. **Breathing:**
   - Inhale as you lift your arms up during the raising phase, drawing air into your lungs and expanding your chest.
   - Exhale as you lower your arms down during the lowering phase, releasing the breath and engaging your core muscles for stability.

Modification Options:

1. **Reduced Range of Motion:**
   - If lifting your arms to shoulder-height is too challenging, you can reduce the range of motion by lifting them to a lower height.

- Start with smaller movements and gradually work your way up to lifting your arms to shoulder-height as you build strength and endurance.

2. **Bent Elbows:**
   - If keeping your arms straight is uncomfortable, you can perform arm raises with slightly bent elbows.
   - This modification reduces strain on the elbow joints while still effectively targeting the muscles of the shoulders and upper back.

Extension Exercises:

1. **Resistance Band Arm Raises:**
   - Hold a resistance band in both hands with your palms facing downwards and your arms relaxed at your sides.
   - Step on the middle of the resistance band with one foot to secure it to the ground.
   - Perform front or side arm raises while holding onto the resistance band, maintaining tension throughout the movement.
   - This adds resistance to the exercise, challenging the muscles of the shoulders and upper back even more.

2. **Weighted Arm Raises:**

   - Hold a light dumbbell or kettlebell in each hand with your palms facing downwards and your arms relaxed at your sides.

   - Perform front or side arm raises while holding onto the weights, maintaining control throughout the movement.

   - The added weight increases the resistance, providing a greater challenge for the muscles of the shoulders and upper back.

3. **Rotating Arm Raises:**

   - Perform front or side arm raises with a rotation at the top of the movement.

   - As you lift your arms, rotate your palms upwards so they face towards the ceiling at the top of the movement.

   - Slowly rotate your palms back downwards as you lower your arms back down to the starting position.

   - This variation adds an additional challenge to the exercise by engaging the muscles of the rotator cuff and increasing shoulder mobility.

Bicep Curls

Bicep curls are a fundamental strength training exercise that targets the muscles of the biceps, forearms, and brachialis. Here are the instructions for performing bicep curls, along with modification options and extension exercises:

1. **Starting Position:**
   - Stand tall with your feet shoulder-width apart, holding a dumbbell in each hand.
   - Let your arms hang naturally at your sides, with your palms facing forward and your elbows close to your body.

2. **Lifting Phase:**
   - Keeping your upper arms stationary, exhale and curl the weights upwards towards your shoulders by bending your elbows.
   - Maintain a controlled and deliberate movement, focusing on contracting your bicep muscles as you lift the weights.
   - Keep your wrists straight throughout the movement, avoiding excessive bending or twisting.

3. **Top Position:**

- Once the dumbbells reach shoulder level or slightly higher, pause briefly to squeeze your biceps at the top of the movement.
  - Focus on fully contracting your biceps and maintaining tension in the muscles.

4. **Lowering Phase:**
  - Inhale and slowly lower the dumbbells back down to the starting position, straightening your elbows and returning to the initial position.
  - Resist the urge to let the weights drop quickly, and maintain control throughout the lowering phase.

5. **Breathing:**
  - Exhale as you lift the weights upwards during the lifting phase, engaging your core muscles and focusing on your biceps.
  - Inhale as you lower the weights back down during the lowering phase, maintaining stability and control.

Modification Options:

1. **Single Arm Bicep Curls:**

- If using both arms simultaneously is too challenging, you can perform bicep curls one arm at a time.
   - Hold one dumbbell in one hand while keeping the other arm relaxed at your side.
   - Alternate curling each arm while maintaining proper form and control.

2. **Seated Bicep Curls:**
   - Perform bicep curls while seated on a bench or chair to reduce the involvement of your lower body.
   - This modification can help isolate the biceps and prevent cheating by using momentum from the legs.

Extension Exercises:

1. **Hammer Curls:**
   - Hold a dumbbell in each hand with your palms facing inward towards your body, in a neutral grip.
   - Perform bicep curls while keeping your palms facing each other throughout the movement.
   - This variation targets the brachialis muscle in addition to the biceps, providing a well-rounded arm workout.

2. **Concentration Curls:**

- Sit on a bench or chair with your legs spread apart and your feet flat on the ground.
- Hold a dumbbell in one hand and rest your elbow on the inside of your thigh, with your arm fully extended and the weight hanging down towards the floor.
- Perform bicep curls while keeping your upper arm stationary, focusing on fully contracting the bicep at the top of the movement.
- This exercise isolates the biceps and helps improve muscle definition and strength.

3. **Reverse Grip Bicep Curls:**
- Hold a dumbbell in each hand with your palms facing downwards towards the ground.
- Perform bicep curls while keeping your palms facing downwards throughout the movement.
- This variation targets the brachialis and brachioradialis muscles in addition to the biceps, providing a comprehensive arm workout.

Bicep Curls to Shoulder Press

Performing a bicep curl to shoulder press, also known as a "bicep curl and press," is an efficient compound exercise targeting the biceps, shoulders, and triceps. Here are detailed instructions along with modification options and extension exercises:

1. **Starting Position:**
   - Stand with your feet hip-width apart, holding a dumbbell in each hand at arm's length by your sides.
   - Keep your palms facing forward, and maintain a slight bend in your knees to stabilize your lower body.

2. **Bicep Curl:**
   - Begin by performing a bicep curl. Exhale as you bend your elbows and lift the dumbbells towards your shoulders.
   - Keep your upper arms stationary and your wrists straight throughout the movement.
   - Squeeze your biceps at the top of the movement, then slowly lower the dumbbells back down to the starting position while inhaling.

3. **Transition to Shoulder Press:**

- Once you've completed the bicep curl and the dumbbells are near your shoulders, rotate your palms to face forward, preparing for the shoulder press.
   - Press the dumbbells upwards above your head until your arms are fully extended but not locked out.
   - Exhale as you press the weights overhead, engaging your shoulder and tricep muscles.
   - Hold the weights briefly at the top of the movement, maintaining stability and control.

4. **Lowering Phase:**
   - Slowly lower the dumbbells back to shoulder height, returning to the starting position of the shoulder press.
   - Rotate your palms back to the starting position, palms facing forward, and then lower the dumbbells back down to your sides, returning to the starting position of the bicep curl.

5. **Breathing:**
   - Exhale as you lift the dumbbells during both the bicep curl and shoulder press phases.
   - Inhale as you lower the dumbbells during both phases, focusing on controlled movements and maintaining stability.

Modification Options:

1. **Lighter Weights:**
   - If you're new to the exercise or working on form, start with lighter dumbbells until you're comfortable with the movement pattern.
   - Gradually increase the weight as you become stronger and more proficient.

2. **Alternating Arms:**
   - To focus on one arm at a time or to maintain stability, you can alternate arms instead of performing both arms simultaneously.
   - This modification can help address strength imbalances between your arms.

Extension Exercises:

1. **Arnold Press:**
   - Start with the dumbbells at shoulder height, palms facing towards you.
   - Press the dumbbells overhead while rotating your palms outward until they face forward.
   - Lower the dumbbells back down to shoulder height while rotating your palms back towards you.

- This exercise targets the front and side deltoids, as well as the biceps and triceps.

2. **Lateral Raises:**
   - Stand with dumbbells at your sides, palms facing your body.
   - Lift the dumbbells out to the sides until they reach shoulder height.
   - Lower the dumbbells back down with control.
   - This exercise primarily targets the lateral deltoids but also engages the biceps and triceps for stabilization.

3. **Seated Alternating Hammer Curls:**
   - Sit on a bench with a dumbbell in each hand, palms facing inwards towards each other.
   - Alternately curl one dumbbell up towards your shoulder while keeping the other arm stationary.
   - Lower the dumbbell back down with control and repeat on the other side.
   - This exercise targets the biceps and forearms, providing a variation to the traditional bicep curl.

Bicycle Crunches

Bicycle crunches are a highly effective core exercise that targets the rectus abdominis, obliques, and hip flexors while also engaging the lower back muscles. Here are detailed instructions on how to perform bicycle crunches, along with modification options and extension exercises:

1. **Starting Position:**
   - Lie flat on your back on a mat or on the floor with your knees bent and feet flat on the ground.
   - Place your hands behind your head, lightly supporting your head with your fingertips, and keep your elbows pointed out to the sides.
   - Engage your core muscles to press your lower back into the floor and maintain a neutral spine throughout the exercise.

2. **Crunching Movement:**
   - Lift your shoulder blades off the ground, bringing your elbows towards your opposite knee while simultaneously extending the other leg straight out.
   - Rotate your torso and bring your right elbow towards your left knee, while extending your right leg straight out.

- As you crunch, aim to bring your shoulder towards your knee rather than just your elbow, to engage your obliques more effectively.
   - Keep your movements controlled and avoid pulling on your head or neck with your hands.

3. **Bicycle Motion:**
   - Alternate the movement by smoothly and continuously pedaling your legs in a bicycling motion, bringing your opposite elbow towards your opposite knee.
   - Continue this pedaling motion, alternating sides, while keeping your upper body lifted and your core engaged throughout the exercise.

4. **Breathing:**
   - Exhale as you crunch and rotate, bringing your elbow towards your knee, engaging your core muscles fully.
   - Inhale as you return to the starting position, maintaining control and stability.

5. **Repetition:**
   - Aim for a controlled pace, focusing on quality over quantity.

- Perform the exercise for a set number of repetitions or time, gradually increasing as you build strength and endurance.

Modification Options:

1. **Reduced Range of Motion:**
   - If you're new to bicycle crunches or have lower back issues, you can reduce the range of motion by not fully extending your legs or not bringing your shoulder blades as high off the ground.
   - Focus on maintaining proper form and engaging your core muscles throughout the movement.

2. **Bent Knee Variation:**
   - For beginners or those with lower back discomfort, you can perform bicycle crunches with your knees bent at a 90-degree angle instead of fully extending your legs.
   - This modification reduces the strain on the lower back while still effectively targeting the abdominal muscles.

Extension Exercises:

1. **Russian Twists:**

   - Sit on the floor with your knees bent and your feet flat on the ground, holding a weight or medicine ball with both hands.
   - Lean back slightly, engaging your core muscles for stability.
   - Rotate your torso to the right, bringing the weight towards the ground next to your hip, then rotate to the left, bringing the weight towards the ground next to your left hip.
   - Continue alternating sides in a twisting motion, focusing on engaging your obliques.

2. **Plank with Knee to Elbow:**
   - Start in a high plank position with your wrists directly under your shoulders and your body forming a straight line from head to heels.
   - Engage your core muscles and bring your right knee towards your right elbow, rounding your back slightly.
   - Return to the starting plank position and repeat on the other side, bringing your left knee towards your left elbow.
   - Focus on maintaining stability and control throughout the movement, avoiding excessive hip rotation.

3. **Mountain Climbers:**

- Start in a high plank position with your wrists directly under your shoulders and your body forming a straight line from head to heels.

- Engage your core muscles and quickly alternate bringing your knees towards your chest in a running motion.

- Keep your hips low and your movements controlled, maintaining a steady pace throughout the exercise.

Bird Dogs

Bird dogs are a popular core stability exercise that targets the muscles of the lower back, abdominals, and glutes while also improving balance and coordination. Here are detailed instructions on how to perform bird dogs, along with modification options and extension exercises:

1. **Starting Position:**
   - Begin on your hands and knees on a mat or the floor. Align your wrists directly under your shoulders and your knees directly under your hips.
   - Engage your core muscles to maintain a neutral spine, keeping your back flat and your head in line with your spine. Your gaze should be directed towards the floor.

2. **Extension:**
   - Inhale and simultaneously extend your right arm straight out in front of you, parallel to the floor, while also extending your left leg straight back behind you, parallel to the floor.
   - Keep your hips square and avoid rotating your torso or tilting your pelvis to one side.

- Focus on maintaining stability and balance throughout the movement, keeping your core engaged to prevent your lower back from sagging.

3. **Hold:**
   - Hold the extended position briefly, ensuring that your arm, leg, and torso form a straight line from head to heel.
   - Keep your neck relaxed and your gaze towards the floor to maintain proper spinal alignment.

4. **Return to Starting Position:**
   - Exhale as you slowly bring your extended arm and leg back to the starting position, maintaining control and stability throughout the movement.
   - Avoid letting your hand or knee touch the ground before completing the desired number of repetitions.

5. **Alternate Sides:**
   - Repeat the movement on the opposite side, extending your left arm and right leg.
   - Focus on maintaining proper form and control with each repetition, keeping your movements smooth and controlled.

6. **Breathing:**

- Inhale as you extend your arm and leg away from your body, filling your lungs with air and engaging your core muscles.

- Exhale as you return to the starting position, contracting your abdominal muscles and maintaining stability.

Modification Options:

1. **Reduced Range of Motion:**
   - If you're new to bird dogs or have difficulty maintaining stability, you can reduce the range of motion by extending your arm and leg only partially.
   - Focus on maintaining proper form and stability throughout the movement, gradually increasing the range of motion as you become more comfortable.

2. **Static Hold:**
   - If balancing on one arm and leg is too challenging, you can perform a static hold by extending your arm and leg and holding the position without moving.
   - Hold the extended position for a set amount of time, focusing on engaging your core muscles and maintaining stability.

Extension Exercises:

1. **Bird Dog Pulses:**
   - Start in the bird dog position with your right arm and left leg extended.
   - Perform small pulses with your extended arm and leg, moving them slightly up and down while maintaining stability and control.
   - Focus on engaging the muscles of your core and glutes throughout the movement.

2. **Plank with Leg Lift:**
   - Start in a high plank position with your wrists directly under your shoulders and your body forming a straight line from head to heels.
   - Lift one leg off the ground, extending it straight back behind you while keeping your hips level and your core engaged.
   - Hold the extended position briefly, then lower your leg back down and repeat on the opposite side.
   - Focus on maintaining stability and control throughout the movement, avoiding any rotation or sagging in your hips.

3. **Opposite Arm and Leg Lifts:**

- Start in a high plank position with your wrists directly under your shoulders and your body forming a straight line from head to heels.
- Lift your right arm straight out in front of you while simultaneously lifting your left leg straight back behind you.
- Hold the extended position briefly, then lower your arm and leg back down and repeat on the opposite side.
- Focus on maintaining stability and control throughout the movement, engaging your core muscles to prevent any rotation or shifting in your hips.

Boat Pose

Boat pose, also known as Navasana in yoga, is a challenging core-strengthening exercise that targets the abdominal muscles, hip flexors, and lower back. Here are detailed instructions on how to perform boat pose, along with modification options and extension exercises:

1. **Starting Position:**
   - Sit on the floor with your knees bent and your feet flat on the ground, hip-width apart.
   - Place your hands behind your thighs, just above your knees, with your fingertips pointing towards your toes.
   - Lengthen your spine, engage your core muscles, and lift your chest to maintain an upright posture.

2. **Lift Your Legs:**
   - Inhale deeply and lean back slightly as you lift your feet off the ground, bringing your shins parallel to the floor.
   - Keep your knees bent at a 90-degree angle, and balance on your sitting bones while maintaining a straight spine.

3. **Extend Your Arms:**

- Once you feel stable in the lifted position, extend your arms straight out in front of you, parallel to the floor.
  - Keep your palms facing each other, and engage your shoulder blades to keep your chest open and lifted.

4. **Lengthen Through Your Spine:**
  - Lengthen through the crown of your head and reach through your fingertips, creating a straight line from your fingertips to your toes.
  - Keep your gaze forward, focusing on a point in front of you to help maintain balance and stability.

5. **Hold and Breathe:**
  - Hold the boat pose for several breaths, maintaining engagement in your core muscles to support your spine and legs.
  - Take slow, deep breaths in and out through your nose, focusing on maintaining stability and control.

6. **Release and Rest:**
  - To release from boat pose, exhale as you lower your feet back down to the floor, returning to the starting position.
  - Take a moment to rest and reset before repeating the pose for another round.

Modification Options:

1. **Bent Knees Variation:**
   - If straightening your legs is too challenging, you can keep your knees bent throughout the pose.
   - Focus on lifting your chest and engaging your core muscles, even with bent knees, to maintain proper alignment and stability.

2. **Toe Tap Variation:**
   - To reduce the intensity of boat pose, you can lower one foot to the ground at a time, tapping your toes lightly on the floor before lifting them back up.
   - Alternate tapping each foot to the ground while keeping your chest lifted and core engaged.

Extension Exercises:

1. **Dynamic Boat Pose:**
   - From the traditional boat pose position, straighten your legs and extend them forward, maintaining a strong core and lifted chest.

- Inhale as you lean back slightly, lifting your arms overhead and reaching forward, creating a long line from your fingertips to your toes.
- Exhale as you return to the starting position, bringing your knees back in towards your chest and bending your elbows.
- Repeat the movement, flowing smoothly between the extended and bent-knee boat pose variations.

2. **Side-to-Side Boat Pose:**
- Start in the traditional boat pose position with your legs lifted and your arms extended in front of you.
- Inhale deeply and twist your torso to the right, bringing your right hand towards the floor and your left arm towards the ceiling.
- Exhale as you return to the center, then inhale and twist your torso to the left, bringing your left hand towards the floor and your right arm towards the ceiling.
- Continue alternating between the right and left twists, engaging your obliques and core muscles to stabilize and support the movement.

Boxing Punches

Boxing punches are dynamic exercises that engage multiple muscle groups, including the arms, shoulders, chest, core, and legs. Here are detailed instructions on how to perform boxing punches, along with modification options and extension exercises:

1. **Starting Position:**
   - Stand with your feet shoulder-width apart, knees slightly bent, and your core engaged.
   - Bring your fists up to your chin with your elbows bent, and keep your hands in a fist position with your palms facing towards each other.

2. **Jab:**
   - Extend your lead hand (left hand if you're orthodox, right hand if you're southpaw) straight out in front of you, aiming for your target.
   - Keep your wrist straight, rotate your shoulder slightly, and pivot on the ball of your back foot to generate power.
   - Quickly retract your arm back to the starting position after each punch, maintaining a fast and fluid motion.

3. **Cross:**

   - From the starting position, extend your rear hand (right hand if you're orthodox, left hand if you're southpaw) straight out in front of you, crossing your body towards the opposite side.

   - Rotate your hips and shoulders to generate power, and pivot on the ball of your back foot for additional force.

   - Keep your non-punching hand close to your face to protect yourself, and quickly retract your arm back to the starting position after each punch.

4. **Hook:**

   - Bend your elbow to a 90-degree angle and rotate your torso towards the side you're punching with.

   - Swing your lead hand (left hand if you're orthodox, right hand if you're southpaw) in a semi-circular motion, aiming to strike your target from the side.

   - Keep your wrist straight and your elbow in line with your shoulder, and pivot on the ball of your back foot for power.

   - Quickly retract your arm back to the starting position after each punch, maintaining control and speed.

5. **Uppercut:**

- Bend your knees slightly and shift your weight to the side opposite to the hand you're punching with.

- From a low position, drive your rear hand (right hand if you're orthodox, left hand if you're southpaw) upwards in a diagonal motion, aiming to strike your target from below.

- Rotate your hips and shoulders to generate power, and pivot on the ball of your back foot for additional force.

- Quickly retract your arm back to the starting position after each punch, maintaining proper form and technique.

Modification Options:

1. **Reduced Speed/Intensity:**
   - If you're new to boxing or have limitations, you can perform the punches at a slower pace with less force to focus on technique and coordination.
   - Gradually increase the speed and intensity as you become more comfortable with the movements.

2. **Shadow Boxing:**
   - If you don't have access to a punching bag or partner, you can perform boxing punches in the air, focusing on form, speed, and footwork.

- Visualize an opponent in front of you and practice your punches with proper technique and fluidity.

Extension Exercises:

1. **Punching Combinations:**
   - Combine different punches (jabs, crosses, hooks, and uppercuts) into fluid combinations, such as jab-cross-hook or jab-cross-uppercut.
   - Practice transitioning between punches smoothly and efficiently, maintaining balance and control throughout the combination.

2. **Punching Drills:**
   - Set up a timer and perform punching drills for a set duration, alternating between different punches or combinations.
   - Focus on maintaining a consistent rhythm and intensity throughout the drill, challenging your endurance and cardiovascular fitness.

3. **Punching with Resistance:**

- Use resistance bands or hand weights to add resistance to your punches, increasing the challenge and strengthening your arm muscles.

- Maintain proper form and control while punching with resistance, and gradually increase the resistance as you become stronger.

Burpees

Burpees are a dynamic full-body exercise that targets multiple muscle groups while also providing cardiovascular benefits. Here are detailed instructions on how to perform burpees, along with modification options and extension exercises:

1. **Starting Position:**
   - Stand with your feet shoulder-width apart, arms by your sides, and knees slightly bent.
   - Engage your core muscles and maintain a straight back throughout the exercise.

2. **Squat Down:**
   - Lower your body into a squat position by bending your knees and pushing your hips back.
   - Place your hands on the floor in front of you, shoulder-width apart, with your fingers facing forward.

3. **Jump Back into Plank Position:**
   - From the squat position, jump both feet back simultaneously, landing in a plank position with your arms extended.

- Keep your body in a straight line from head to heels, and engage your core muscles to maintain stability.

4. **Push-Up (Optional):**
   - If you want to add an extra challenge, perform a push-up by lowering your chest towards the floor while keeping your elbows close to your body.
   - Push yourself back up to the plank position, maintaining proper form and control throughout the movement.

5. **Jump Forward into Squat Position:**
   - Jump both feet forward towards your hands, returning to the squat position with your hands on the floor.
   - Use the momentum from the jump to propel yourself back into the starting position.

6. **Jump Upwards:**
   - Explode upwards into a vertical jump, reaching your arms overhead.
   - Land softly on the balls of your feet and immediately lower back down into the squat position to begin the next repetition.

7. **Repeat:**

- Continue performing the sequence of movements in a fluid motion for the desired number of repetitions or time.

Modification Options:

1. **Step Back Instead of Jumping:**
   - Instead of jumping both feet back into the plank position, step one foot back at a time to reduce impact and intensity.
   - Step forward one foot at a time to return to the squat position before jumping upwards.

2. **Elevated Surface for Hands:**
   - If reaching the floor is challenging, perform burpees with your hands placed on an elevated surface such as a bench, chair, or step.
   - This modification reduces the range of motion required for the push-up portion of the exercise.

Extension Exercises:

1. **Burpee Variations:**
   - Experiment with different variations of burpees, such as adding a tuck jump at the top of the movement or

incorporating a burpee box jump by jumping onto a box or platform instead of straight up.

   - You can also try burpee pull-ups by adding a pull-up at the top of the movement.

2. **Burpee Ladder:**

   - Perform a ladder workout by increasing or decreasing the number of burpees in each set.

   - For example, start with 10 burpees, then 9, then 8, and so on, until you reach 1 burpee per set, or vice versa.

3. **Weighted Burpees:**

   - Hold a pair of dumbbells or a weighted vest while performing burpees to increase the resistance and challenge your muscles further.

   - Start with lighter weights and gradually increase the resistance as you become stronger and more proficient.

Butt Kicks

Butt kicks are a dynamic cardiovascular exercise that targets the quadriceps, hamstrings, and calves while also improving lower body flexibility and coordination. Here are detailed instructions on how to perform butt kicks, along with modification options and extension exercises:

1. **Starting Position:**
   - Stand tall with your feet hip-width apart and your arms by your sides.
   - Engage your core muscles to maintain stability and keep your back straight throughout the exercise.

2. **Running Motion:**
   - Begin by jogging in place at a slow to moderate pace, lifting your feet off the ground and bringing your heels towards your glutes with each step.
   - Aim to kick your heels up towards your buttocks, alternating between your left and right legs in a running motion.

3. **Increase Speed:**

- Gradually increase the pace of the movement, pumping your arms rhythmically in coordination with your legs.
   - Strive for a quick and controlled motion, focusing on bringing your heels towards your glutes with each step.

4. **Maintain Form:**
   - Keep your upper body tall and your shoulders relaxed throughout the exercise.
   - Avoid leaning forward or backward, and maintain a natural stride length as you jog in place.

5. **Breathing:**
   - Breathe steadily and rhythmically throughout the exercise, inhaling and exhaling in sync with your movements.
   - Aim to maintain a consistent breathing pattern to support your cardiovascular endurance.

6. **Duration:**
   - Continue performing butt kicks for a set duration, such as 30 seconds to 1 minute, or for a specific number of repetitions.
   - Gradually increase the duration or intensity of the exercise as you build strength and endurance.

Modification Options:

1. **Reduced Impact:**
   - If the impact of jogging in place is too intense, you can perform butt kicks at a slower pace or with less force.
   - Focus on lifting your heels towards your glutes in a controlled manner, rather than aiming for speed.

2. **Low-Impact Variation:**
   - Perform a low-impact version of butt kicks by stepping one foot back at a time, bringing your heel towards your glute in a controlled motion.
   - This modification reduces the impact on your joints while still engaging the muscles of the lower body.

Extension Exercises:

1. **High Knees with Butt Kicks:**
   - Combine butt kicks with high knees to create a dynamic cardio workout.
   - Alternate between bringing your knees up towards your chest and kicking your heels towards your glutes in a continuous motion.

2. **Interval Training:**
   - Incorporate butt kicks into a high-intensity interval training (HIIT) workout by alternating between periods of maximum effort and rest.
   - Perform butt kicks at maximum intensity for 20-30 seconds, followed by a 10-20 second rest period, and repeat for multiple rounds.

3. **Skipping Variation:**
   - Perform butt kicks while skipping in place, alternating between kicking your heels towards your glutes and hopping lightly on the balls of your feet.
   - This variation adds an extra challenge to the exercise and increases coordination and agility.

Calf Raises

Calf raises are an effective exercise for targeting the calf muscles, specifically the gastrocnemius and soleus. Here are detailed instructions on how to perform calf raises, along with modification options and extension exercises, including calf raises with pulses:

1. **Starting Position:**
   - Stand tall with your feet hip-width apart, and your arms hanging naturally by your sides.
   - Engage your core muscles to maintain balance and stability throughout the exercise.

2. **Lift Heels:**
   - Slowly lift your heels off the ground as high as you can, rising onto the balls of your feet.
   - Keep your weight centered over the balls of your feet and avoid rolling onto the outer edges or inner edges of your feet.

3. **Squeeze Calves:**

- Hold the raised position at the top for a brief moment, focusing on squeezing your calf muscles to maximize the contraction.
   - Aim to lift your heels as high as possible without compromising your balance or form.

4. **Lower Heels:**
   - Slowly lower your heels back down to the starting position, allowing your heels to gently touch the ground.
   - Maintain control throughout the lowering phase to prevent bouncing or jerking movements.

5. **Repeat:**
   - Perform the calf raises for the desired number of repetitions, aiming for a smooth and controlled motion with each repetition.
   - Focus on maintaining proper form and technique throughout the exercise.

Modification Options:

1. **Wall Calf Raises:**
   - Stand with your hands resting lightly against a wall for support.

   - Perform calf raises as described, using the wall for stability if needed, especially if you're new to the exercise or working on balance.

2. **Seated Calf Raises:**
   - Sit on a chair or bench with your feet flat on the ground and your knees bent at a 90-degree angle.
   - Place a weight (such as a dumbbell) on your thighs just above your knees for added resistance.
   - Lift your heels off the ground as high as you can, then lower them back down in a controlled manner.

3. **Single-Leg Calf Raises:**
   - Perform calf raises on one leg at a time to isolate and strengthen each calf individually.
   - Lift one foot off the ground and balance on the other foot while performing the calf raises.

4. **Assisted Calf Raises:**
   - Hold onto a stable surface, such as a wall or countertop, for support and balance while performing calf raises.
   - This modification can help you focus on proper form and technique without worrying about balance.

Extension Exercises:

1. **Calf Raises with Pulse:**
   - Perform a regular calf raise as described, but instead of lowering your heels all the way down, pause at the bottom position and then lift your heels slightly off the ground again.
   - Pulse up and down in this bottom range of motion for several repetitions before completing the full range of motion.

2. **Calf Raises on a Step:**
   - Stand on the edge of a step or sturdy platform with your heels hanging off the edge.
   - Lower your heels down below the level of the step, then lift them as high as you can above the level of the step.
   - This exercise allows for a greater range of motion and can help to increase the stretch and activation of the calf muscles.

3. **Calf Raise Jumps:**
   - Start in the raised position of a calf raise with your heels lifted off the ground.
   - Explosively push off the balls of your feet and jump into the air as high as possible.

- Land softly back onto the balls of your feet and immediately transition into another calf raise.

Cat-Cow Stretch

The Cat-Cow Stretch is a gentle yoga exercise that helps to improve flexibility and mobility in the spine while also stretching the back, chest, and shoulders. Here are detailed instructions on how to perform the Cat-Cow Stretch, along with modification options and extension exercises:

1. **Starting Position (Neutral Spine):**
   - Begin on your hands and knees in a tabletop position, with your wrists directly under your shoulders and your knees under your hips.
   - Keep your spine in a neutral position, with your back flat and your neck in line with your spine.

2. **Cow Pose (Extension):**
   - As you inhale, arch your back and lift your chest towards the ceiling, allowing your belly to sink towards the floor.
   - Lift your tailbone towards the ceiling and tilt your pelvis slightly forward.
   - Gaze upwards or towards the ceiling, opening up your chest and shoulders.

3. **Cat Pose (Flexion):**

- As you exhale, round your spine towards the ceiling, tucking your chin towards your chest.
- Press firmly into the ground with your hands and knees, engaging your abdominal muscles as you draw your belly button towards your spine.
- Allow your head to release towards the floor, creating a gentle stretch in the back of your neck.

4. **Flow Between Poses:**
- Flow smoothly between Cow Pose and Cat Pose, moving with your breath.
- Inhale as you transition into Cow Pose, arching your back and lifting your chest.
- Exhale as you transition into Cat Pose, rounding your spine and tucking your chin.
- Continue flowing between the two poses for several breaths, moving at a pace that feels comfortable for you.

5. **Repeat:**
- Repeat the Cat-Cow Stretch for several rounds, focusing on the fluid movement of your spine and breath.

Modification Options:

1. **Reduced Range of Motion:**
   - If you have limited flexibility in your spine or experience discomfort, reduce the range of motion in each pose.
   - Instead of arching deeply into Cow Pose or rounding deeply into Cat Pose, focus on moving within a comfortable range that allows you to feel a gentle stretch without strain.

2. **Support for Wrists:**
   - If you have wrist discomfort, place a folded towel or yoga mat under your wrists for additional support.
   - You can also perform the Cat-Cow Stretch on fists or using yoga blocks to decrease pressure on the wrists.

Extension Exercises:

1. **Extended Cat-Cow Stretch:**
   - After moving through several rounds of the traditional Cat-Cow Stretch, add a side bend to each pose.
   - In Cow Pose, reach one arm towards the ceiling while maintaining the arch in your back, creating a side stretch along the torso.
   - In Cat Pose, thread one arm under the opposite arm, bringing your shoulder and ear towards the ground for a side stretch on the other side of the body.

- Alternate between these variations on each round, flowing with your breath.

2. **Child's Pose to Cat-Cow Flow:**
   - Begin in Child's Pose, sitting back on your heels with your arms extended in front of you and your forehead resting on the mat.
   - From Child's Pose, transition into Cat Pose by rounding your spine and pressing into your hands to lift your hips towards the ceiling.
   - Flow smoothly into Cow Pose by arching your back and lifting your chest, then return to Child's Pose to complete the cycle.
   - Move with your breath, flowing between Child's Pose, Cat Pose, and Cow Pose for several rounds.

Chair Dips

Chair dips are a great bodyweight exercise for targeting the muscles of the triceps, shoulders, and chest. Here are detailed instructions on how to perform chair dips, along with modification options and extension exercises:

1. **Starting Position:**
   - Sit on the edge of a sturdy chair or bench with your hands gripping the front edge of the seat, fingers pointing towards your body.
   - Place your feet flat on the ground in front of you, knees bent at a 90-degree angle, and your back close to the edge of the chair.

2. **Lower Your Body:**
   - Slowly slide your buttocks off the edge of the chair while keeping your hands gripping the seat.
   - Lower your body towards the floor by bending your elbows, allowing them to flare out to the sides.
   - Keep your back close to the chair and your elbows pointing directly behind you, rather than out to the sides.

3. **Maintain Control:**

- Lower your body until your elbows are bent at approximately a 90-degree angle or slightly less, feeling a stretch in your triceps.
   - Keep your shoulders down and back, and avoid letting your shoulders hunch up towards your ears.
   - Maintain control throughout the movement, avoiding any sudden or jerky motions.

4. **Push Back Up:**
   - Press into the palms of your hands to straighten your arms and lift your body back up to the starting position.
   - Fully extend your arms at the top of the movement, but avoid locking your elbows to maintain tension in the triceps.
   - Keep your core engaged throughout the exercise to stabilize your body and prevent excessive swinging or leaning.

5. **Repeat:**
   - Perform the desired number of repetitions, aiming for a smooth and controlled motion with each dip.
   - Focus on maintaining proper form and technique throughout the exercise.

Modification Options:

1. **Partial Range of Motion:**
   - If performing full chair dips is too challenging, start by performing partial range of motion dips.
   - Lower your body only partway down towards the floor, focusing on maintaining control and stability in the shoulders and elbows.
   - Gradually increase the depth of the dips as you build strength and confidence.

2. **Assisted Chair Dips:**
   - Place your feet on the floor further away from the chair to decrease the intensity of the exercise.
   - The further your feet are from the chair, the less weight you'll be lifting, making the exercise easier.
   - You can also perform assisted chair dips by using a resistance band looped around the chair and under your knees for support.

Extension Exercises:

1. **Triceps Kickbacks:**

- Hold a dumbbell in each hand and hinge forward at the hips, keeping your back flat and your arms extended towards the floor.
   - Bend your elbows to bring the weights up towards your shoulders, then extend your arms straight back behind you, focusing on squeezing the triceps.
   - Slowly lower the weights back down to the starting position and repeat for several repetitions.

2. **Triceps Push-Ups:**
   - Start in a high plank position with your hands directly under your shoulders and your body forming a straight line from head to heels.
   - Lower your body towards the floor by bending your elbows, keeping them close to your sides.
   - Push back up to the starting position, fully extending your arms.
   - Focus on keeping your core engaged and your body in a straight line throughout the movement.

Child's Pose

Child's Pose is a relaxing yoga pose that stretches the back, shoulders, hips, and thighs while promoting relaxation and stress relief. Here are detailed instructions on how to perform Child's Pose, along with modification options and extension exercises:

1. **Starting Position:**
   - Begin on your hands and knees in a tabletop position, with your wrists directly under your shoulders and your knees under your hips.
   - Take a moment to find a comfortable and stable position, with your spine in a neutral alignment.

2. **Sit Back:**
   - On an exhale, slowly lower your hips back towards your heels, bringing your forehead to rest on the mat.
   - Keep your arms extended in front of you, palms facing down, and your fingertips reaching forward.
   - Allow your chest to gently sink towards the floor, lengthening through your spine.

3. **Open Hips:**

- Spread your knees apart wide, allowing your torso to sink down between your thighs.
   - If it's comfortable, you can also bring your big toes to touch behind you, creating a wider stretch in the hips.

4. **Relax and Breathe:**
   - Close your eyes if it feels comfortable, and focus on deepening your breath.
   - Take slow, deep breaths into your belly, allowing your body to relax and soften with each exhale.
   - Stay in Child's Pose for several breaths or as long as feels comfortable, allowing tension to release from your body.

5. **Release:**
   - To come out of the pose, gently walk your hands back towards your body, lifting your torso back up to a tabletop position.
   - Sit back on your heels for a moment and notice how your body feels after the stretch.

Modification Options:

1. **Supported Child's Pose:**

- If you have difficulty sitting back on your heels or reaching your forehead to the mat, place a folded blanket or cushion between your buttocks and heels for support.
   - You can also place a cushion or yoga block under your forehead to support your head and neck.

2. **Knee Support:**
   - If you have discomfort in your knees, place a folded towel or blanket under your knees for additional cushioning.
   - Adjust the width of your knees as needed to find a comfortable position that allows you to relax into the pose.

Extension Exercises:

1. **Thread the Needle:**
   - From Child's Pose, extend your right arm towards the right side, threading it under your left arm.
   - Rest your right shoulder and ear on the mat, and gently twist your torso to the left.
   - Hold the stretch for several breaths, feeling a deep stretch in the right shoulder and upper back.
   - Repeat on the other side by extending your left arm towards the left side and threading it under your right arm.

2. **Extended Child's Pose Variation:**
   - From Child's Pose, walk your hands over to one side of the mat, stretching through the side of your body.
   - Hold the stretch for several breaths, feeling a deep stretch along the side of your torso and through the arm.
   - Repeat on the other side by walking your hands over to the opposite side of the mat.

Dead Bug

Dead Bug is a core-strengthening exercise that targets the abdominal muscles while also improving stability and coordination. Here are detailed instructions on how to perform Dead Bug, along with modification options and extension exercises, including Dead Bug with Ball Squeeze:

1. **Starting Position:**
   - Lie on your back on a mat with your arms extended towards the ceiling, directly above your shoulders.
   - Bend your knees and hips to a 90-degree angle, with your shins parallel to the floor.
   - Engage your core muscles to press your lower back into the mat and maintain a neutral spine.

2. **Arm and Leg Movement:**
   - Begin by simultaneously lowering your right arm and left leg towards the floor, keeping them hovering just above the ground.
   - Keep your core engaged and your lower back pressed into the mat to stabilize your spine.
   - Maintain control throughout the movement, avoiding any arching or rounding of the back.

3. **Return to Starting Position:**

   - Slowly return your right arm and left leg to the starting position, bringing them back to the ceiling.

   - Keep your movements controlled and deliberate, focusing on engaging the abdominal muscles.

4. **Alternate Sides:**

   - Repeat the movement on the opposite side, lowering your left arm and right leg towards the floor while keeping them hovering just above the ground.

   - Again, focus on maintaining stability in your core and pelvis throughout the movement.

5. **Continue Alternating:**

   - Alternate between lowering your arms and legs, moving in a controlled and coordinated manner.

   - Aim to keep your movements smooth and fluid, maintaining tension in the abdominal muscles throughout the exercise.

Modification Options:

1. **Partial Range of Motion:**

- If lowering both arms and legs simultaneously is too challenging, you can start by lowering one arm or one leg at a time.
   - Gradually increase the difficulty by lowering both limbs simultaneously as you build strength and stability.

2. **Bent Knee Variation:**
   - If you have lower back discomfort or difficulty maintaining a neutral spine, you can perform Dead Bug with your knees bent instead of straight.
   - Start with your knees bent at a 90-degree angle and follow the same arm and leg movement pattern described above.

Extension Exercises:

1. **Dead Bug with Ball Squeeze:**
   - Hold a small exercise ball or cushion between your knees throughout the Dead Bug movement.
   - As you lower your arms and legs towards the floor, squeeze the ball gently between your knees to engage the inner thigh muscles.

- This variation adds an extra challenge for the core and lower body muscles, as you'll need to maintain stability while also squeezing the ball.

2. **Straight Leg Dead Bug:**
   - Once you've mastered the basic Dead Bug movement, you can progress to the straight leg variation.
   - Instead of bending your knees to 90 degrees, keep your legs straight as you lower them towards the floor.
   - This variation increases the demand on the core muscles and requires greater stability to control the movement.

Fast Feet

Fast feet, also known as quick feet or agility drills, are a dynamic exercise that improves foot speed, agility, and coordination. Here are detailed instructions on how to perform fast feet, along with modification options and extension exercises:

1. **Starting Position:**
   - Begin by standing with your feet shoulder-width apart and your knees slightly bent.
   - Keep your arms bent at a 90-degree angle, elbows close to your sides, and hands in loose fists.

2. **Rapid Movement:**
   - Quickly alternate moving your feet up and down, tapping the balls of your feet on the ground as fast as you can.
   - Keep your movements light and springy, minimizing the time your feet spend on the ground with each tap.
   - Focus on maintaining a quick pace and rhythm throughout the exercise.

3. **Stay on the Balls of Your Feet:**

- Keep your weight centered over the balls of your feet, with your heels lightly lifted off the ground.
   - Avoid letting your heels touch the ground as you tap your feet, as this slows down the movement and reduces the effectiveness of the exercise.

4. **Arms Movement:**
   - Coordinate the movement of your arms with your feet, swinging them back and forth in sync with your foot taps.
   - Keep your elbows bent at a 90-degree angle and your hands relaxed as you swing your arms.

5. **Maintain Control:**
   - Focus on maintaining control and coordination throughout the exercise, even as you pick up the pace.
   - Keep your core engaged to stabilize your body and prevent excessive movement in the upper body.

6. **Duration:**
   - Perform fast feet for a set duration, such as 30 seconds to 1 minute, or for a specific number of repetitions.
   - Gradually increase the duration or intensity of the exercise as you become more proficient.

Modification Options:

1. **Slow Down the Pace:**
   - If performing fast feet at a rapid pace is too challenging, start by slowing down the movement.
   - Focus on tapping your feet on the ground at a comfortable pace, gradually increasing the speed as you build confidence and coordination.

2. **Reduce Range of Motion:**
   - If maintaining a full range of motion with your feet is difficult, focus on smaller, quicker movements.
   - Instead of lifting your feet as high off the ground, focus on tapping the ground with the balls of your feet while keeping your movements fast and controlled.

Extension Exercises:

1. **Agility Ladder Drills:**
   - Set up an agility ladder on the ground and perform various footwork drills, such as high knees, lateral shuffles, or crossover steps.
   - Use the agility ladder to improve foot speed, agility, and coordination through a variety of dynamic movements.

2. **Box Jumps:**

   - Stand in front of a sturdy box or platform and jump onto it explosively, landing softly with both feet.

   - Step or jump back down to the starting position and repeat for multiple repetitions, focusing on quick and powerful movements.

3. **Sprint Intervals:**

   - Incorporate fast feet into sprint intervals by performing quick feet drills for a set duration followed by a short sprint.

   - Alternate between periods of fast feet and sprinting to improve speed, agility, and cardiovascular fitness.

Flutter Kicks

Flutter kicks are an effective core exercise that targets the lower abdominal muscles and hip flexors while also improving stability and endurance. Here are detailed instructions on how to perform flutter kicks, along with modification options and extension exercises:

1. **Starting Position:**
   - Lie flat on your back on a mat with your arms by your sides and your palms pressing into the floor.
   - Engage your core muscles to press your lower back into the mat and maintain a neutral spine.
   - Lift your legs off the ground a few inches, keeping them straight and together.

2. **Fluttering Movement:**
   - Begin by alternately kicking your legs up and down in a quick and controlled motion.
   - Keep your legs straight and toes pointed throughout the movement.
   - Aim to maintain a steady and even pace, focusing on engaging the lower abdominal muscles.

3. **Maintain Control:**
   - Avoid letting your legs drop too low towards the ground, as this can strain the lower back.
   - Keep your movements controlled and within a comfortable range of motion, focusing on engaging the core muscles.

4. **Breathing:**
   - Breathe steadily and rhythmically throughout the exercise, inhaling and exhaling in sync with your leg movements.
   - Avoid holding your breath, and aim to maintain a consistent breathing pattern to support your effort.

5. **Duration:**
   - Perform flutter kicks for a set duration, such as 30 seconds to 1 minute, or for a specific number of repetitions.
   - Gradually increase the duration or intensity of the exercise as you become more proficient.

Modification Options:

1. **Reduced Range of Motion:**

- If lifting both legs off the ground is too challenging, you can perform flutter kicks with one leg at a time.
   - Keep one leg extended straight while the other leg rests on the ground, alternating between legs in a fluttering motion.
   - This modification reduces the demand on the core muscles while still engaging the lower abdominal muscles and hip flexors.

2. **Bent Knee Variation:**
   - If you have difficulty keeping your legs straight, you can perform flutter kicks with your knees slightly bent.
   - This variation reduces strain on the lower back and allows you to focus on engaging the core muscles effectively.

Extension Exercises:

1. **Scissor Kicks:**
   - After completing a set of flutter kicks, transition into scissor kicks by crossing one leg over the other in a scissoring motion.
   - Alternate between crossing one leg over the other in a controlled and fluid movement, focusing on engaging the lower abdominal muscles.

2. **Leg Raises:**

   - Transition from flutter kicks into leg raises by lifting both legs straight up towards the ceiling.

   - Lower your legs back down towards the ground without letting them touch, then lift them back up to complete one repetition.

   - Focus on maintaining control and stability throughout the movement, engaging the core muscles to lift and lower the legs.

3. **Weighted Flutter Kicks:**

   - Hold a light dumbbell or medicine ball between your feet while performing flutter kicks to increase the resistance and challenge the core muscles further.

   - Start with a light weight and gradually increase the resistance as you become stronger and more proficient.

Flyes

Performing flyes without weights can still effectively engage the chest muscles and improve muscular endurance. Here are detailed instructions on how to perform bodyweight flyes, along with modification options and extension exercises:

1. **Starting Position:**
   - Lie flat on your back on a mat with your knees bent and feet planted firmly on the ground.
   - Extend your arms out to the sides with palms facing up, creating a "T" shape with your body.

2. **Engage Your Core:**
   - Engage your core muscles to stabilize your spine and maintain a neutral position throughout the exercise.
   - Keep your shoulder blades pulled down and back to prevent them from lifting off the ground.

3. **Lowering Phase:**
   - Slowly bring your arms together in a wide arc motion, crossing them over your chest towards the midline of your body.

- Focus on engaging the chest muscles as you bring your arms together, feeling a stretch across your chest.

4. **Stretch Position:**
   - Pause briefly at the bottom of the movement, feeling the stretch in your chest muscles.
   - Maintain control and avoid bouncing or jerking the movement to prevent injury.

5. **Lifting Phase:**
   - Contract your chest muscles to bring your arms back to the starting position, reversing the movement in a controlled manner.
   - Focus on squeezing your chest muscles at the top of the movement to maximize the contraction.

6. **Breathing:**
   - Inhale as you lower your arms towards the midline of your body, and exhale as you bring them back to the starting position.
   - Focus on breathing rhythmically and steadily throughout the exercise to support your effort and maintain proper form.

7. **Repetition:**

- Perform bodyweight flyes for the desired number of repetitions, focusing on quality over quantity and maintaining proper form throughout.

Modification Options:

1. **Bench Angle:**
   - Adjust the angle of the bench to target different areas of the chest.
   - Performing flyes on an incline bench targets the upper chest, while performing them on a decline bench targets the lower chest.

2. **Arm Position:**
   - Experiment with different arm positions to target different areas of the chest.
   - Bringing your arms together in front of your chest targets the inner chest, while bringing them together slightly above chest level targets the mid-chest.

Extension Exercises:

1. **Reverse Flyes without Weights:**

- Stand with your feet hip-width apart and hinge forward at the hips, keeping your back flat and chest lifted.
   - Extend your arms straight down towards the ground with palms facing each other.
   - Lift your arms out to the sides in a wide arc motion until they are parallel to the ground, squeezing your shoulder blades together at the top of the movement.
   - Lower your arms back towards the starting position with control and repeat.

2. **Reverse Flyes with Dumbbells:**
   - Hold a pair of light dumbbells in each hand and hinge forward at the hips, keeping your back flat and chest lifted.
   - Extend your arms straight down towards the ground with palms facing each other.
   - Lift the dumbbells out to the sides in a wide arc motion until your arms are parallel to the ground, squeezing your shoulder blades together at the top of the movement.
   - Lower the dumbbells back towards the starting position with control and repeat.

3. **Bent Over Reverse Flyes:**
   - Stand with your feet hip-width apart and hold a pair of light dumbbells in each hand.

- Hinge forward at the hips, keeping your back flat and chest lifted, until your torso is parallel to the ground.

- Extend your arms straight down towards the ground with palms facing each other.

- Lift the dumbbells out to the sides in a wide arc motion until your arms are parallel to the ground, squeezing your shoulder blades together at the top of the movement.

- Lower the dumbbells back towards the starting position with control and repeat.

Fold Forward

Forward fold, also known as Uttanasana in yoga, is a rejuvenating pose that stretches the hamstrings, calves, and spine while promoting relaxation and stress relief. Here are detailed instructions on how to perform forward fold, along with modification options and extension exercises, including forward fold with quad stretch and seated forward fold:

1. **Starting Position:**
   - Begin standing tall with your feet hip-width apart and your arms by your sides.
   - Take a moment to ground yourself, feeling the connection between your feet and the earth beneath you.

2. **Hinge at the Hips:**
   - On an exhale, slowly begin to hinge forward at the hips, keeping your spine long and your back flat.
   - Bend forward from the hips rather than rounding your back, maintaining a slight bend in your knees to avoid strain.

3. **Reach for Your Feet:**
   - Allow your hands to hang down towards the floor, reaching for your feet or the backs of your ankles.

- If you're unable to reach your feet, you can place your
hands on your shins or thighs instead.

4. **Relax Your Neck:**
   - Release any tension in your neck and shoulders, allowing
your head to hang heavy towards the floor.
   - Keep a gentle gaze towards your knees or shins to avoid
straining your neck.

5. **Breathe and Relax:**
   - Take slow, deep breaths into your belly, allowing your
body to relax and soften with each exhale.
   - Feel the stretch along the back of your legs and spine,
breathing into any areas of tension or tightness.

6. **Hold the Pose:**
   - Hold the forward fold for several breaths, allowing gravity
to gently deepen the stretch.
   - Focus on relaxing into the pose and surrendering to the
sensation of the stretch.

Modification Options:

1. **Bent Knees Variation:**

- If you have tight hamstrings or lower back discomfort, you can perform forward fold with bent knees.

- Bend your knees generously to allow your torso to fold forward comfortably while still maintaining a long spine.

2. **Use Props for Support:**

- Place yoga blocks or a folded blanket on the floor beneath your hands to provide support and lift if you're unable to reach the ground.

- This modification helps to maintain proper alignment and prevents straining.

Extension Exercises:

1. **Forward Fold with Quad Stretch:**

- From standing, bend your right knee and reach back with your right hand to grasp the top of your right foot or ankle.

- As you exhale, hinge forward at the hips, folding your torso towards your left leg while keeping your right knee bent.

- Feel the stretch in the quadriceps of your right leg as you fold forward. Hold for several breaths, then switch sides.

2. **Seated Forward Fold (Paschimottanasana):**

- Sit on the floor with your legs extended straight in front of you and your feet flexed towards your body.

- On an exhale, hinge forward at the hips, reaching for your feet or shins with your hands.

- Keep your spine long and your chest lifted as you fold forward, feeling the stretch along the backs of your legs.

- Hold the pose for several breaths, breathing deeply into the stretch.

Glute Bridges

Glute bridges are a great exercise for strengthening the glutes, hamstrings, and lower back muscles while also improving hip stability and mobility. Here are detailed instructions on how to perform glute bridges, along with modification options and extension exercises, including glute bridge marches:

1. **Starting Position:**
   - Lie flat on your back on a mat with your knees bent and your feet flat on the floor, hip-width apart.
   - Keep your arms by your sides, palms facing down, and engage your core muscles to stabilize your spine.

2. **Lift Your Hips:**
   - On an exhale, press through your heels to lift your hips towards the ceiling, squeezing your glutes at the top of the movement.
   - Keep your upper back and shoulders on the mat, focusing on using your glutes to lift your hips rather than pushing through your lower back.

3. **Full Extension:**

- Aim to lift your hips as high as possible without overarching your lower back or straining your neck.

- Pause at the top of the movement for a brief moment to fully engage your glutes before lowering back down.

4. **Lower with Control:**

- Slowly lower your hips back down to the starting position, maintaining control throughout the movement.

- Avoid dropping your hips too quickly or bouncing at the bottom of the movement.

5. **Repeat:**

- Perform the glute bridges for the desired number of repetitions, focusing on maintaining proper form and engaging the glutes with each repetition.

Modification Options:

1. **Single-Leg Glute Bridges:**

- If you're looking to increase the challenge or address muscle imbalances, you can perform single-leg glute bridges.

- Lift one foot off the ground and extend it straight out in front of you, then perform the glute bridge movement with the other leg.
   - Keep your hips level and your core engaged throughout the exercise.

2. **Elevated Glute Bridges:**
   - Place your feet on an elevated surface, such as a bench or sturdy chair, to increase the range of motion and intensity of the exercise.
   - This modification targets the glutes and hamstrings more intensely while also engaging the core for stability.

Extension Exercises:

1. **Glute Bridge Marches:**
   - Perform a standard glute bridge, lifting your hips towards the ceiling and squeezing your glutes at the top of the movement.
   - While maintaining the bridge position, lift one foot off the ground and bring your knee towards your chest, then lower it back down.

- Alternate between lifting each leg in a marching motion while keeping your hips stable and level throughout the movement.
   - Focus on engaging the glutes and maintaining proper form, avoiding any rocking or twisting of the hips.

2. **Weighted Glute Bridges:**
   - Hold a dumbbell or kettlebell on your hips to add resistance to the glute bridge movement.
   - This variation increases the intensity of the exercise and helps to build strength and muscle mass in the glutes and hamstrings.

Incorporate glute bridges into your lower body workout routine to strengthen the glutes, hamstrings, and lower back muscles, and improve hip stability and mobility. Experiment with different modification options and extension exercises to tailor the exercise to your individual needs and goals, gradually progressing as you become stronger and more proficient.

High Knees

High knees are a dynamic cardiovascular exercise that engages the lower body muscles, improves coordination, and boosts heart rate. Here are detailed instructions on how to perform high knees, along with modification options and extension exercises, including high knees with a twist:

1. **Starting Position:**
   - Stand tall with your feet hip-width apart and your arms hanging naturally by your sides.
   - Engage your core muscles to stabilize your spine and maintain good posture throughout the exercise.

2. **Lift Your Knees:**
   - Begin by lifting your right knee towards your chest as high as you can while simultaneously bringing your left arm forward, elbow bent at a 90-degree angle.
   - Keep your foot flexed and your toes pointing towards your shin to engage the hip flexors and drive the movement.

3. **Alternate Sides:**

- Lower your right leg back down to the ground as you simultaneously lift your left knee towards your chest, bringing your right arm forward.
   - Continue alternating between lifting your knees in a running motion, driving your arms in sync with your legs.

4. **Pace and Intensity:**
   - Aim to perform the high knees at a quick pace, driving your knees up as fast as you can while maintaining control and proper form.
   - Focus on lifting your knees high towards your chest with each repetition to maximize the engagement of the hip flexors and core muscles.

5. **Breathing:**
   - Breathe rhythmically throughout the exercise, inhaling and exhaling in sync with your movements.
   - Avoid holding your breath, and focus on maintaining a steady breathing pattern to support your effort.

Modification Options:

1. **Reduced Impact:**

- If high-impact movements are challenging or uncomfortable, you can perform a modified version of high knees with a lower intensity.
- Instead of lifting your knees as high, focus on marching in place, lifting each knee towards hip level without hopping or jumping.

2. **Slow Pace:**
   - If performing high knees at a fast pace is too challenging, you can slow down the movement and focus on lifting your knees with control.
   - Gradually increase the speed as you build strength and endurance.

Extension Exercises:

1. **High Knees with Twist:**
   - Perform high knees as described above, but add a twisting motion to engage the obliques and further challenge the core muscles.
   - As you lift each knee towards your chest, twist your torso slightly towards the lifted knee, bringing the opposite elbow towards the knee.

- Alternate between twisting towards each knee with each repetition, maintaining a quick pace and driving the movement with your arms and legs.

2. **High Knee Sprints:**
   - Perform high knees at a maximum intensity, driving your knees up as fast as you can while maintaining proper form.
   - Aim to cover a short distance as quickly as possible, focusing on driving your arms and lifting your knees high with each stride.
   - This variation increases the cardiovascular challenge and helps to improve speed and agility.

Jump Rope

Jumping rope is a fantastic cardiovascular exercise that improves coordination, agility, and endurance while burning calories and strengthening muscles. Here are detailed instructions on how to perform jump rope, along with modification options and extension exercises:

1. **Choose the Right Rope:**
   - Select a jump rope that is the appropriate length for your height. Stand on the middle of the rope and adjust the handles so they reach your armpits.
   - Use a lightweight speed rope for faster rotations and a heavier rope for more resistance.

2. **Proper Form:**
   - Hold the handles of the jump rope in each hand with palms facing forward.
   - Start with the rope behind you and rotate it over your head and down towards the ground in a circular motion.
   - As the rope approaches your feet, jump off the ground using the balls of your feet.

3. **Jumping Technique:**

- Jump only high enough to clear the rope, about 1 to 2 inches off the ground.
- Land softly on the balls of your feet, keeping your knees slightly bent to absorb the impact.
- Maintain a straight posture with your shoulders back and your core engaged throughout the exercise.

4. **Rope Rotation:**
- Use your wrists, not your arms, to rotate the jump rope. Keep your elbows close to your sides and your forearms parallel to the ground.
- Rotate the rope quickly and smoothly, allowing it to pass under your feet with each jump.

5. **Breathing:**
- Breathe rhythmically throughout the exercise, inhaling through your nose as you prepare to jump and exhaling through your mouth as you jump.

6. **Practice and Persistence:**
- Start with short sessions of jumping rope, gradually increasing the duration as you become more comfortable and proficient.

- Focus on maintaining a consistent rhythm and pace, striving for smooth and controlled movements.

Modification Options:

1. **Single Leg Jumps:**
   - Practice jumping rope on one leg at a time, alternating between left and right legs.
   - This modification helps improve balance, coordination, and ankle stability.

2. **Double Unders:**
   - Perform two rotations of the jump rope for every jump, requiring greater speed and coordination.
   - Start by mastering regular jumps before attempting double unders.

Extension Exercises:

1. **High Knees with Jump Rope:**
   - Perform high knees while jumping rope, lifting your knees as high as possible with each jump.
   - This variation increases the intensity of the exercise and further engages the core and leg muscles.

2. **Cross Over Jumps:**
   - Cross the jump rope in front of your body with each jump, alternating the direction of the cross with each rotation.
   - This variation challenges coordination and agility while adding a dynamic twist to the exercise.

3. **Jump Rope Intervals:**
   - Incorporate jump rope intervals into your workout routine, alternating between periods of jumping rope and other exercises such as bodyweight exercises or strength training.
   - This variation adds variety to your workout and helps to improve cardiovascular fitness and endurance.

Jumping Jacks

Jumping jacks are a classic cardiovascular exercise that engages multiple muscle groups while elevating heart rate. Here are detailed instructions on how to perform jumping jacks, along with modification options and extension exercises:

1. **Starting Position:**
   - Stand tall with your feet together and your arms by your sides.
   - Maintain good posture with your shoulders back and core engaged.

2. **Jumping Motion:**
   - Jump into the air, spreading your legs out to the sides while simultaneously raising your arms above your head.
   - Keep your arms straight and your palms facing each other as you reach overhead.
   - Land softly on the balls of your feet with your legs wider than hip-width apart and your arms extended.

3. **Return to Starting Position:**

- Jump back to the starting position by bringing your feet together and lowering your arms back down to your sides.
   - Keep a fluid and controlled motion throughout the exercise, maintaining a steady pace.

4. **Repetition:**
   - Continue performing jumping jacks for the desired number of repetitions or for a set duration.

Modification Options:

1. **Low-Impact Variation:**
   - If the impact of traditional jumping jacks is too intense, you can perform a low-impact variation by stepping instead of jumping.
   - Step to the side with one foot while simultaneously raising your arms overhead, then return to the starting position and repeat on the opposite side.

2. **Reduced Range of Motion:**
   - If you have limited mobility or joint discomfort, you can reduce the range of motion by performing smaller movements.

- Bend your knees slightly and raise your arms to shoulder height instead of overhead while performing the jumping motion.

Extension Exercises:

1. **Jumping Jacks with Cross:**
   - Perform traditional jumping jacks, but add a cross in front of your body with your arms.
   - As you jump and spread your legs, cross your arms in front of your chest, alternating which arm is on top with each repetition.
   - This variation engages the chest and shoulders more intensely while adding a dynamic twist to the exercise.

2. **Jumping Jacks with Squat:**
   - Combine jumping jacks with squats to increase the intensity and engage the lower body muscles further.
   - Perform a squat as you jump your feet out to the sides, then return to standing as you bring your feet together and raise your arms overhead.
   - Focus on maintaining proper squat form with your knees tracking over your toes and your chest lifted throughout the movement.

3. **Speed Variation:**

   - Increase the speed of your jumping jacks to elevate your heart rate and challenge your cardiovascular fitness.

   - Perform jumping jacks as quickly as you can while maintaining proper form, focusing on moving with agility and coordination.

Leg Raises

Leg raises are an effective exercise for targeting the abdominal muscles, particularly the lower abdominals, while also engaging the hip flexors and lower back muscles. Here are detailed instructions on how to perform leg raises, along with modification options and extension exercises:

1. **Starting Position:**
   - Lie flat on your back on a mat with your arms by your sides and your palms pressing into the floor.
   - Engage your core muscles to press your lower back into the mat and maintain a neutral spine throughout the exercise.

2. **Raise Your Legs:**
   - Begin by lifting both legs off the ground simultaneously, keeping them straight and together.
   - Use your abdominal muscles to lift your legs towards the ceiling, aiming to bring them perpendicular to the floor.

3. **Controlled Lowering:**
   - Slowly lower your legs back down towards the ground, maintaining control and resisting gravity.

- Avoid letting your feet touch the ground completely, keeping them hovering just above the floor to maintain tension in the abdominal muscles.

4. **Avoid Arching the Back:**
   - Keep your lower back pressed into the mat throughout the movement to avoid arching and strain on the spine.
   - Focus on using your abdominal muscles to control the movement rather than relying on momentum.

5. **Breathing:**
   - Exhale as you lift your legs towards the ceiling, and inhale as you lower them back down towards the ground.
   - Focus on breathing rhythmically throughout the exercise to support your effort and engage the core muscles effectively.

6. **Repetition:**
   - Perform leg raises for the desired number of repetitions, focusing on quality over quantity and maintaining proper form throughout.

Modification Options:

1. **Bent Knee Leg Raises:**
   - If lifting both legs straight is too challenging or causes lower back discomfort, you can perform bent knee leg raises instead.
   - Bend your knees and lift them towards your chest, keeping your feet together and your shins parallel to the floor.
   - Focus on engaging the lower abdominal muscles to lift your knees towards your chest while keeping your lower back pressed into the mat.

2. **Partial Range of Motion:**
   - If you're unable to lift your legs all the way to perpendicular, you can perform leg raises with a reduced range of motion.
   - Focus on lifting your legs as high as you can while maintaining control and proper form, gradually increasing the range of motion as you become stronger.

Extension Exercises:

1. **Flutter Kicks:**

- After completing a set of leg raises, transition into flutter kicks by lowering your legs slightly towards the ground and alternating lifting one leg up while lowering the other.
   - Keep your legs straight and your movements quick and controlled, focusing on engaging the lower abdominal muscles.

2. **Hanging Leg Raises:**
   - If you have access to a pull-up bar or hanging apparatus, you can perform hanging leg raises to increase the challenge.
   - Hang from the bar with an overhand grip and lift your legs towards the ceiling, keeping them straight and together.
   - Lower your legs back down with control, avoiding swinging or using momentum to lift your legs.

Lunges

Lunges are a versatile lower body exercise that targets multiple muscle groups, including the quadriceps, hamstrings, glutes, and calves. Here are detailed instructions on how to perform lunges, along with modification options and extension exercises:

1. **Starting Position:**
   - Stand tall with your feet hip-width apart and your arms by your sides.
   - Engage your core muscles to stabilize your spine and maintain good posture throughout the exercise.

2. **Step Forward:**
   - Take a big step forward with your right foot, landing heel-first.
   - Lower your body towards the ground by bending both knees, keeping your torso upright and your chest lifted.

3. **Lowering Motion:**
   - Lower your body until your front thigh is parallel to the ground, and your back knee is hovering just above the floor.

- Keep your front knee aligned with your ankle and avoid letting it extend past your toes.

4. **Push Back:**
   - Push through the heel of your front foot to return to the starting position, driving your body back up to standing.
   - Keep your movements controlled and avoid locking out your knees at the top of the movement.

5. **Repeat on Other Side:**
   - Perform the same movement with your left leg, stepping forward into a lunge and then returning to the starting position.

Modification Options:

1. **Reverse Lunges:**
   - Instead of stepping forward, step backward into the lunge motion.
   - This variation reduces strain on the knees and may be more accessible for beginners.

2. **Lateral Lunges:**

- Step to the side with your right foot, bending your right knee and lowering your body towards the ground.
   - Return to the starting position and repeat on the left side.
   - This variation targets the inner and outer thighs and adds variety to your workout.

Extension Exercises:

1. **Jumping Lunges:**
   - From a standing position, jump into a lunge with your right foot forward and your left foot back.
   - Quickly switch legs in mid-air, landing with your left foot forward and your right foot back.
   - Continue alternating legs with each jump, maintaining a rapid pace.
   - This variation adds a cardiovascular element and increases the intensity of the exercise.

2. **Walking Lunges:**
   - Take a large step forward with your right foot and lower into a lunge.
   - Push through your right heel to return to standing and immediately step forward into a lunge with your left foot.

- Continue alternating legs and moving forward with each lunge.
   - This variation challenges balance and coordination while also providing a dynamic leg workout.

3. **Reverse Lunges with Front Kick:**
   - Perform a reverse lunge by stepping backward with your right foot and lowering into a lunge position.
   - As you return to standing, drive your right knee up towards your chest and extend your leg forward into a front kick.
   - Return to the starting position and repeat on the left side.
   - This variation targets the quadriceps, glutes, and hip flexors while also engaging the core and improving balance.

4. **Curtsy Lunges:**
   - Step your right foot diagonally behind your left leg, crossing it behind your body as if performing a curtsy.
   - Lower your body into a lunge position, keeping your chest lifted and your knees aligned.
   - Push through the heel of your left foot to return to standing and repeat on the other side.
   - This variation targets the glutes and outer thighs while also engaging the quadriceps and hamstrings.

5. **Side Lunges with Knee Drive:**

   - Step to the right with your right foot, bending your right knee and lowering your body towards the ground.

   - Push through your right heel to return to standing and lift your left knee towards your chest.

   - Lower your left foot back to the ground and repeat on the left side.

   - This variation targets the inner and outer thighs, glutes, and hip flexors while also improving balance and stability.

Mountain Climber

Mountain climbers are a dynamic full-body exercise that primarily targets the core muscles while also engaging the upper body and lower body muscles. Here are detailed instructions on how to perform mountain climbers, along with modification options and extension exercises, including mountain climber with a twist:

1. **Starting Position:**
   - Begin in a plank position with your hands directly under your shoulders and your body forming a straight line from head to heels.
   - Engage your core muscles to stabilize your spine and keep your hips level throughout the exercise.

2. **Drive the Knees:**
   - Lift your right foot off the ground and bring your right knee towards your chest, keeping your toes pointed.
   - As you return your right foot to the starting position, simultaneously drive your left knee towards your chest in a fluid motion.
   - Alternate between driving each knee towards your chest in a running motion, maintaining a quick pace.

3. **Maintain Proper Form:**
   - Keep your shoulders stacked over your wrists and your arms straight throughout the exercise.
   - Avoid sagging your hips or lifting them too high, aiming to maintain a straight line from head to heels.
   - Focus on engaging the core muscles to drive the movement and prevent excessive rocking or swaying.

4. **Breathe Rhythmically:**
   - Coordinate your breathing with your movements, inhaling as you extend your legs back and exhaling as you drive your knees towards your chest.
   - Focus on breathing steadily and rhythmically throughout the exercise to support your effort and engage the core muscles effectively.

5. **Repetition:**
   - Continue performing mountain climbers for the desired number of repetitions or for a set duration, maintaining a quick and controlled pace.

Modification Options:

1. **Reduced Speed:**
   - If performing mountain climbers at a quick pace is too challenging, you can slow down the movement and focus on maintaining proper form.
   - Perform the exercise at a pace that allows you to maintain control and engage the core muscles effectively.

2. **Elevated Surface:**
   - Place your hands on an elevated surface, such as a bench or step, to reduce the demand on the core muscles and make the exercise more accessible.
   - This modification allows you to focus on proper form and gradually increase the intensity as you become stronger.

Extension Exercises:

1. **Mountain Climber with Twist:**
   - Perform mountain climbers as described above, but add a twist to engage the obliques and further challenge the core muscles.
   - As you drive each knee towards your chest, rotate your hips and bring your knee towards the opposite elbow, crossing the body.

- Alternate between twisting to the left and right with each repetition, maintaining a quick pace and fluid motion.

2. **Cross-Body Mountain Climbers:**
   - Instead of driving your knees towards your chest, aim to bring each knee towards the opposite elbow in a cross-body motion.
   - This variation targets the obliques and improves coordination while also engaging the core muscles and increasing the intensity of the exercise.

Oblique Crunches

Oblique crunches and their variations into your core workout routine to strengthen and tone the oblique muscles, improve core stability, and enhance overall posture. Here are detailed instructions on how to perform oblique crunches, along with modification options and extension exercises, including standing oblique crunches:

1. **Starting Position:**
   - Lie on your back with your knees bent and feet flat on the floor.
   - Place your hands lightly behind your head, elbows pointing out to the sides, or cross your arms over your chest.

2. **Engage Your Core:**
   - Engage your abdominal muscles by drawing your belly button towards your spine to stabilize your torso.

3. **Crunch to the Side:**
   - Lift your shoulder blades off the floor and rotate your torso to one side, bringing your elbow towards your opposite knee.

  - Focus on contracting the oblique muscles on the side of your torso as you perform the crunch.

4. **Squeeze and Hold:**
  - Pause briefly at the top of the movement, feeling the contraction in your obliques.
  - Keep your movements controlled and avoid using momentum to swing your body.

5. **Return to Starting Position:**
  - Slowly lower your shoulder blades back down to the floor, returning to the starting position.
  - Repeat the crunch on the same side for the desired number of repetitions before switching to the other side.

6. **Alternate Sides:**
  - Perform an equal number of repetitions on each side, maintaining proper form and control throughout the exercise.

Modification Options:

1. **Bent-Knee Oblique Crunches:**

- If you find it challenging to keep your legs straight, you can perform the crunches with your knees bent and feet flat on the floor.
  - This modification reduces the leverage and makes the exercise more accessible for beginners.

2. **Reduce Range of Motion:**
  - If you're new to oblique crunches or have limited flexibility, you can reduce the range of motion by performing smaller crunches.
  - Focus on contracting the oblique muscles while maintaining proper alignment of the spine and torso.

Extension Exercises:

1. **Standing Oblique Crunches:**
  - Stand with your feet shoulder-width apart and place your hands lightly behind your head.
  - Crunch your torso to one side, bringing your elbow towards your hip while lifting the opposite knee towards the elbow.
  - Focus on contracting the oblique muscles on the side of your torso as you perform the standing crunch.

- Repeat the crunches on both sides for the desired number of repetitions, maintaining proper form and control throughout.

2. **Side Plank Oblique Crunches:**
   - Start in a side plank position with your body in a straight line from head to heels, resting on one forearm and the side of one foot.
   - Place your top hand lightly behind your head and bring your top elbow towards your bottom hip, performing a crunch.
   - Focus on contracting the oblique muscles on the underside of your torso as you perform the crunch.
   - Repeat the crunches on both sides for the desired number of repetitions, maintaining proper form and control throughout.

Plank

Plank is a fundamental core exercise that targets multiple muscle groups, including the abdominals, obliques, and lower back. Here are detailed instructions on how to perform plank, along with modification options and extension exercises:

1. **Starting Position:**
   - Begin by kneeling on the floor with your hands placed directly under your shoulders.
   - Extend your legs behind you and rise up onto your toes, creating a straight line from your head to your heels.
   - Engage your core muscles to stabilize your spine and prevent your hips from sagging or lifting too high.

2. **Hold Position:**
   - Maintain the plank position, keeping your body aligned and your muscles engaged.
   - Focus on breathing steadily and deeply, avoiding holding your breath.

3. **Form Check:**

   - Ensure that your shoulders are stacked directly over your wrists and your elbows are slightly bent.

   - Keep your neck in line with your spine, avoiding any strain or tension in the neck muscles.

   - Maintain a strong and stable core by bracing your abdominals and drawing your belly button towards your spine.

4. **Hold Time:**

   - Aim to hold the plank position for a set duration, gradually increasing the time as you become stronger and more comfortable with the exercise.

   - Start with shorter holds, such as 20-30 seconds, and gradually progress to longer durations.

Modification Options:

1. **Knee Plank:**

   - If the full plank position is too challenging, you can perform a knee plank by resting on your knees instead of your toes.

   - Maintain the same alignment and form as the full plank position, engaging your core muscles and keeping your body in a straight line from your head to your knees.

2. **Forearm Plank:**
   - Lower down onto your forearms instead of placing your hands directly under your shoulders.
   - Keep your elbows stacked under your shoulders and your forearms parallel to each other.
   - This modification reduces strain on the wrists and may be more comfortable for some individuals.

Extension Exercises:

1. **High Plank with Shoulder Taps:**
   - From the full plank position, lift one hand off the ground and tap your opposite shoulder.
   - Return your hand to the starting position and repeat on the other side, alternating between shoulder taps while maintaining a stable core.

2. **Plank Jacks:**
   - Start in the full plank position and jump both feet out to the sides, then back together.
   - Keep your core engaged and your hips stable throughout the movement, focusing on maintaining proper form.

3. **Plank Up-Downs:**

   - Begin in the full plank position on your hands.

   - Lower down onto your right forearm, followed by your left forearm, then press back up onto your right hand and left hand.

   - Repeat the movement, alternating which arm you lower down with first.

4. **Plank with Alternating Arm Reach:**

   - From the full plank position, extend your right arm forward, reaching it out in front of you.

   - Return your right hand to the starting position and repeat with your left arm, alternating between reaching each arm forward while maintaining a stable core.

5. **Plank with Arm and Leg Lift:**

   - Lift your right arm and left leg off the ground, reaching them out in front of you and behind you, respectively.

   - Return to the starting position and repeat with your left arm and right leg, alternating between lifting opposite limbs while keeping your hips level.

6. **Plank with Hip Dips:**

- From the full plank position, rotate your hips to the right, lowering them towards the ground.
  - Return to the starting position and repeat on the left side, alternating between dipping your hips to each side while maintaining a stable core.

7. **Plank with Knee to Elbow:**
  - From the full plank position, draw your right knee towards your right elbow, crunching your obliques.
  - Return to the starting position and repeat on the left side, alternating between bringing each knee towards the opposite elbow.

8. **Plank with Leg Lifts:**
  - Lift your right leg off the ground, keeping it straight and engaging your glutes and hamstrings.
  - Lower your right leg back down and repeat with your left leg, alternating between lifting each leg while maintaining a stable core.

9. **Plank with Shoulder Taps and Leg Lifts:**
  - Combine the movements of high plank with shoulder taps and plank with leg lifts, alternating between tapping each

shoulder and lifting each leg while keeping your core engaged and stable.

10. **Side Planks:**
   - Start in the full plank position and rotate your body to the right, balancing on your right hand and the outer edge of your right foot.
   - Keep your body in a straight line from head to heels, engaging your obliques to maintain stability.
   - Hold the side plank position for a set duration, then repeat on the left side.

11. **Side Planks with Leg Lift:**
   - From the side plank position, lift your top leg towards the ceiling, engaging your glutes and outer thigh muscles.
   - Lower your leg back down and repeat, focusing on maintaining stability in the side plank position while lifting your leg.

12. **Side Plank with Rotation:**
   - Start in the side plank position on your right side, with your left hand placed on

your hip or extended towards the ceiling.

- Rotate your torso towards the floor, bringing your left arm underneath your body.

- Return to the starting position and repeat, focusing on engaging your obliques and maintaining stability throughout the movement.

Pushup

Push-ups are a classic bodyweight exercise that primarily target the chest, shoulders, and triceps while also engaging the core and back muscles. Here are detailed instructions on how to perform push-ups, along with modification options and extension exercises:

1. **Starting Position:**
   - Begin in a high plank position with your hands slightly wider than shoulder-width apart and your wrists aligned under your shoulders.
   - Extend your legs behind you, with your feet hip-width apart and toes pressing into the ground.
   - Engage your core muscles to maintain a straight line from your head to your heels, avoiding any sagging or arching in the lower back.

2. **Lowering Phase:**
   - Bend your elbows and lower your chest towards the ground, keeping your elbows close to your body at a 45-degree angle.
   - Lower yourself until your chest nearly touches the ground, maintaining a controlled and steady movement.

3. **Pushing Phase:**
   - Press through your palms and extend your arms to push yourself back up to the starting position.
   - Keep your body in a straight line throughout the movement, avoiding any excessive movement or rotation.

4. **Breathing:**
   - Inhale as you lower your body towards the ground, and exhale as you push yourself back up to the starting position.
   - Focus on maintaining a steady and controlled breathing pattern throughout the exercise.

5. **Repetition:**
   - Perform push-ups for the desired number of repetitions, aiming for quality over quantity and focusing on maintaining proper form throughout.

Modification Options:

1. **Knee Push-ups:**
   - If performing push-ups from the toes is too challenging, you can perform knee push-ups instead.

- Start in a high plank position with your knees resting on the ground and your body forming a straight line from your head to your knees.
   - Lower your chest towards the ground by bending your elbows, then push yourself back up to the starting position.

2. **Elevated Surface Push-ups:**
   - Place your hands on an elevated surface, such as a bench or step, to reduce the intensity of the push-up.
   - Keep your body in a straight line from head to heels and perform the push-up as you would from the floor.

Extension Exercises:

1. **Diamond Push-ups:**
   - Place your hands close together directly under your chest, forming a diamond shape with your thumbs and index fingers.
   - Perform push-ups with your hands in this narrow position to target the triceps and inner chest muscles.

2. **Push-ups with Shoulder Taps:**
   - Perform a push-up, then at the top of the movement, lift one hand off the ground and tap the opposite shoulder.

   - Return your hand to the starting position and repeat on the other side, alternating between shoulder taps while maintaining a stable core.

3. **Wide Grip Push-ups:**
   - Place your hands wider than shoulder-width apart to target the chest muscles from a different angle.
   - Perform push-ups with your hands in this wide position, focusing on maintaining proper form and engaging the chest muscles throughout the movement.

4. **Tricep Push-ups:**
   - Position your hands close together directly under your chest, with your elbows pointing back towards your feet.
   - Lower your body towards the ground, keeping your elbows close to your sides to target the triceps muscles.

5. **Push-up to Side Plank:**
   - Perform a push-up, then at the top of the movement, rotate your body to the left and extend your left arm towards the ceiling into a side plank position.
   - Return to the starting position and repeat on the other side, alternating between push-ups and side planks to engage the core and shoulder stabilizers.

Rows

Performing rows without weights can effectively engage the back muscles and improve strength and endurance. Here are detailed instructions on how to perform bodyweight rows, along with modification options and extension exercises:

1. **Set Up:**
   - Find a sturdy horizontal bar or surface that is about waist height, such as a table edge, railing, or low bar in a gym.
   - Lie underneath the bar facing up, positioning yourself so that your body is straight and your heels are on the ground.

2. **Grip the Bar:**
   - Reach up and grab the bar with an overhand grip (palms facing away from you) or an underhand grip (palms facing towards you), slightly wider than shoulder-width apart.
   - Keep your arms fully extended and your body in a straight line from head to heels.

3. **Pull Yourself Up:**
   - Engage your back muscles and pull your chest towards the bar by bending your elbows and squeezing your shoulder blades together.

- Focus on initiating the movement from your back muscles
rather than your arms, keeping your elbows close to your
body.

4. **Squeeze and Lower:**
   - Once your chest reaches the bar, pause briefly and
squeeze your back muscles at the top of the movement.
   - Slowly lower yourself back down to the starting position
with control, maintaining tension in your back muscles
throughout the movement.

5. **Breathing:**
   - Inhale as you lower yourself down towards the ground,
and exhale as you pull yourself up towards the bar.
   - Focus on breathing rhythmically and steadily throughout
the exercise to support your effort and maintain proper form.

6. **Repetition:**
   - Perform bodyweight rows for the desired number of
repetitions, focusing on quality over quantity and maintaining
proper form throughout.

Modification Options:

1. **Foot Position:**

   - Adjust the difficulty of the exercise by changing the angle of your body.

   - To make the exercise easier, walk your feet closer to the bar so that your body is at a more upright angle.

   - To increase the challenge, walk your feet further away from the bar so that your body is at a more horizontal angle.

2. **Grip Width:**

   - Experiment with different grip widths to target different areas of the back.

   - A wider grip emphasizes the upper back and rear deltoids, while a narrower grip targets the mid-back and biceps.

Extension Exercises:

1. **Dumbbell Rows:**

   - Stand with your feet shoulder-width apart and hold a dumbbell in each hand with palms facing each other.

   - Hinge forward at the hips, keeping your back flat and chest lifted, until your torso is parallel to the ground.

   - Pull the dumbbells up towards your sides by bending your elbows and squeezing your shoulder blades together.

- Lower the dumbbells back towards the starting position with control and repeat.

2. **Bent Over Rows with Dumbbells:**
   - Stand with your feet shoulder-width apart and hold a dumbbell in each hand with palms facing towards your body.
   - Hinge forward at the hips, keeping your back flat and chest lifted, until your torso is almost parallel to the ground.
   - Pull the dumbbells up towards your sides by bending your elbows and squeezing your shoulder blades together.
   - Lower the dumbbells back towards the starting position with control and repeat.

Russian Twists

Russian twists are an effective exercise for targeting the obliques and improving rotational core strength. Here are detailed instructions on how to perform Russian twists, along with modification options and extension exercises:

1. **Starting Position:**
   - Sit on the floor with your knees bent and feet flat on the ground, keeping your back straight and chest lifted.
   - Lean back slightly to engage your core muscles and create a V-shape with your torso and thighs.

2. **Hand Position:**
   - Hold a weight or medicine ball with both hands, positioning it in front of your chest.
   - Alternatively, you can clasp your hands together or keep them in a prayer position in front of your chest.

3. **Twisting Motion:**
   - Engage your core muscles and rotate your torso to the right, bringing the weight or hands towards the floor next to your right hip.

- Keep your chest lifted and avoid rounding your back as you twist.

   - Pause briefly at the bottom of the movement, feeling the contraction in your obliques.

4. **Return to Center:**
   - Reverse the twisting motion and rotate your torso to the left, bringing the weight or hands towards the floor next to your left hip.

   - Maintain control throughout the movement and avoid swinging or using momentum to twist.

5. **Breathing:**
   - Inhale as you rotate your torso to one side, and exhale as you return to the center and rotate to the other side.

   - Focus on breathing rhythmically and steadily throughout the exercise to support your effort and engage the core muscles effectively.

6. **Repetition:**
   - Perform Russian twists for the desired number of repetitions or time, focusing on quality over quantity and maintaining proper form throughout.

Modification Options:

1. **Bodyweight Russian Twists:**
   - Perform Russian twists without holding any weight, focusing on engaging the core muscles and maintaining proper form throughout the movement.
   - This modification reduces the intensity of the exercise and is suitable for beginners or those with limited equipment.

2. **Feet Supported Russian Twists:**
   - Sit on the floor with your knees bent and feet elevated off the ground, resting on a bench or stable surface.
   - Engage your core muscles to maintain balance and stability throughout the movement, focusing on rotating your torso from side to side.

Extension Exercises:

1. **Russian Twist with Leg Extension:**
   - Perform a Russian twist as described above, holding a weight or keeping your hands clasped together in front of your chest.
   - As you rotate your torso to one side, extend your legs out straight in front of you, hovering them off the ground.

- Bring your legs back towards the starting position as you return to the center, then repeat on the other side.

- This variation increases the challenge by adding a lower body component to the exercise, engaging the hip flexors and lower abdominals.

2. **Russian Twist with Reach:**

- Perform a Russian twist as described above, holding a weight or keeping your hands clasped together in front of your chest.

- As you rotate your torso to one side, reach the weight or hands towards the floor next to your hip, extending your arm fully.

- Return to the center and then repeat on the other side, reaching towards the opposite hip.

- This variation increases the range of motion and engages the shoulders and upper back muscles in addition to the core and obliques.

Seated Spinal Twist

Seated spinal twists are beneficial for improving spinal mobility and flexibility, as well as stretching the muscles along the spine and in the hips. Here are detailed instructions on how to perform seated spinal twists, along with modification options and extension exercises:

1. **Starting Position:**
   - Sit on the floor with your legs extended straight out in front of you.
   - Sit up tall with a straight spine, and engage your core muscles to support your lower back.

2. **Leg Position:**
   - Bend your right knee and cross your right foot over your left leg, placing it flat on the floor outside your left thigh.
   - Keep your left leg extended and toes pointing up towards the ceiling.

3. **Hand Placement:**
   - Place your left hand on the outside of your right knee, providing gentle pressure to deepen the twist.

- Keep your right hand on the floor behind you for support, fingertips pointing towards your spine.

4. **Twisting Motion:**
   - Inhale as you lengthen your spine and lift your chest towards the ceiling.
   - Exhale as you gently twist your torso to the right, using your left hand on your right knee to deepen the stretch.
   - Keep your hips grounded and both sit bones evenly pressing into the floor.

5. **Head Position:**
   - Turn your head to look over your right shoulder, keeping your chin parallel to the floor.
   - Avoid straining your neck or forcing the twist beyond your comfortable range of motion.

6. **Breathing:**
   - Maintain steady, deep breathing throughout the stretch, inhaling to lengthen the spine and exhaling to deepen the twist.
   - Focus on relaxing into the stretch with each exhale, allowing your body to gradually release tension.

7. **Hold and Release:**
   - Hold the twist for 15-30 seconds, feeling a gentle stretch along the spine and in the muscles of the back and hips.
   - To release, slowly unwind the twist on an exhale, returning to the starting position with both legs extended.

8. **Repeat on the Other Side:**
   - Switch the position of your legs, bending your left knee and crossing your left foot over your right leg.
   - Repeat the same twisting motion to the left side, placing your right hand on the outside of your left knee and twisting your torso to the left.

Modification Options:

1. **Chair Modification:**
   - If sitting on the floor is uncomfortable, you can perform seated spinal twists in a chair.
   - Sit towards the front edge of a sturdy chair with your feet flat on the ground and knees bent at 90-degree angles.
   - Follow the same instructions for the twisting motion, using the backrest of the chair for support as needed.

2. **Gentle Variation:**

- If you have limited flexibility or mobility in the spine, you can perform a gentler version of the twist.
   - Sit up tall with your legs extended straight out in front of you, and simply twist your torso to one side without using your hands to deepen the stretch.
   - Hold the twist for a few breaths, then return to the center and repeat on the other side.

Extension Exercises:

1. **Seated Spinal Twist with Bind:**
   - Once you're comfortable with the basic seated spinal twist, you can add a bind to deepen the stretch.
   - After twisting your torso, reach your left hand behind your back and your right hand under your right thigh, clasping your hands together if possible.
   - Use the bind to gently deepen the twist and open up the chest and shoulders.

2. **Seated Spinal Twist with Forward Fold:**
   - After holding the seated spinal twist on each side, add a forward fold to stretch the back and hamstrings.
   - Extend both legs straight out in front of you and hinge forward at the hips, reaching your hands towards your feet.

- Keep your spine long and chest lifted as you fold forward, feeling a stretch along the entire length of the spine.

Seated Toe Touches

Seated toe touches are excellent for stretching the hamstrings, lower back, and improving overall flexibility. Here are detailed instructions on how to perform seated toe touches, along with modification options and extension exercises:

1. **Starting Position:**
   - Sit on the floor with your legs extended straight out in front of you, toes pointing up towards the ceiling.
   - Sit up tall with a straight spine, engaging your core muscles to support your lower back.

2. **Reach Towards Your Toes:**
   - Inhale deeply, lengthening your spine and lifting your chest towards the ceiling.
   - Exhale as you hinge forward at the hips, leading with your chest and reaching your hands towards your toes.
   - Keep your back flat and avoid rounding your spine as you fold forward.

3. **Maintain Length in the Spine:**

   - Focus on keeping your spine long and your chest lifted throughout the movement.

   - Imagine reaching your heart towards your toes rather than collapsing over your legs.

4. **Flexibility Limitation:**

   - Only go as far as you comfortably can while maintaining good form.

   - You may not be able to touch your toes initially, and that's okay. Focus on the stretch sensation in the back of your legs.

5. **Hold and Breathe:**

   - Hold the stretch for 15-30 seconds, breathing deeply and allowing your muscles to relax and release tension.

   - Keep your breath slow and steady, inhaling through your nose and exhaling through your mouth.

6. **Return to Starting Position:**

   - On an inhale, slowly lift your torso back up to the starting position, stacking each vertebra one on top of the other.

   - Take a moment to reset and reestablish proper posture before repeating the stretch.

7. **Repeat:**
   - Repeat the stretch for 2-3 sets, focusing on smooth, controlled movements and gradually increasing your range of motion over time.

Modification Options:

1. **Bent Knee Toe Touches:**
   - If you have tight hamstrings or limited flexibility, you can perform toe touches with bent knees.
   - Bend your knees slightly and perform the same forward fold motion, reaching your hands towards your feet or ankles.

2. **Use a Strap or Towel:**
   - If you can't reach your toes comfortably, you can use a yoga strap or towel to assist you.
   - Loop the strap around the soles of your feet and hold onto the ends, using it to gently pull yourself forward into the stretch.

Extension Exercises:

1. **Seated Forward Fold with Side Stretch:**

- After performing seated toe touches, add a side stretch to target the obliques and side body.
   - Sit up tall with your legs extended in front of you and your arms reaching overhead.
   - Exhale as you hinge forward at the hips, reaching your hands towards your toes.
   - Once you're in the forward fold, walk your hands over to one side, feeling a stretch along the opposite side of your torso.
   - Hold the stretch for 15-30 seconds, then return to the center and repeat on the other side.

2. **Seated Forward Fold with Spinal Twist:**
   - Perform a seated forward fold as described above, reaching your hands towards your toes.
   - Once you're in the forward fold, place your right hand on the ground behind you and twist your torso to the left, reaching your left arm up towards the ceiling.
   - Hold the stretch for 15-30 seconds, feeling a gentle twist through your spine, then return to the center and repeat on the other side.

Shoulder Presses

Performing a bodyweight shoulder press is an effective way to strengthen the shoulder muscles and improve upper body stability. Here are detailed instructions on how to perform a bodyweight shoulder press, along with modification options and extension exercises:

1. **Starting Position:**
   - Stand with your feet shoulder-width apart and your arms bent at 90 degrees, elbows pointing down towards the ground.
   - Engage your core muscles to stabilize your spine and keep your torso upright.

2. **Hand Position:**
   - Position your hands slightly wider than shoulder-width apart, with palms facing forward.
   - Your fingertips should be pointing towards the ceiling, and your elbows should be in line with your shoulders.

3. **Pressing Motion:**
   - Exhale as you press your arms overhead, straightening your elbows and extending your arms fully.

   - Keep your core engaged and avoid arching your lower
back as you press the arms overhead.

4. **Full Extension:**
   - Fully extend your arms overhead, reaching towards the
ceiling with your fingertips.
   - Focus on keeping your shoulders down away from your
ears and maintaining stability through your core and lower
body.

5. **Controlled Lowering:**
   - Inhale as you slowly lower your arms back to the starting
position, bending your elbows to return to the 90-degree
angle.
   - Maintain control throughout the movement, resisting the
urge to drop your arms quickly.

6. **Repetition:**
   - Perform the bodyweight shoulder press for the desired
number of repetitions, focusing on quality over quantity and
maintaining proper form throughout.

Modification Options:

1. **Seated Shoulder Press:**
   - Perform the shoulder press while seated on a stable chair or bench.
   - This modification reduces the stability challenge and allows you to focus more on isolating the shoulder muscles.

2. **Assisted Shoulder Press:**
   - Stand with your back against a wall for stability support.
   - Perform the shoulder press as described above, using the wall for support and balance assistance if needed.

Extension Exercises:

1. **Shoulder Press with Dumbbells:**
   - Hold a dumbbell in each hand with palms facing forward, and perform the shoulder press as described above.
   - This variation adds resistance to the exercise, allowing you to progressively overload the shoulder muscles for strength gains.

2. **Alternating Shoulder Press:**
   - Hold a dumbbell in each hand with palms facing forward, and start with your arms bent at 90 degrees.

- Press one arm overhead while keeping the other arm bent at 90 degrees.

- Lower the first arm back down as you press the opposite arm overhead, alternating sides with each repetition.

Side Leg Raises

Side leg raises are an effective exercise for targeting the muscles of the outer thighs (abductors) and hips, helping to improve lower body strength and stability. Here are detailed instructions on how to perform side leg raises, along with modification options and extension exercises:

1. **Starting Position:**
   - Lie on your side on a mat with your legs stacked on top of each other.
   - Prop yourself up on your bottom elbow to support your upper body, or lay your head on your bottom arm for comfort.
   - Engage your core muscles to stabilize your spine and pelvis throughout the exercise.

2. **Leg Position:**
   - Keep your top leg straight and in line with your body, with toes pointing forward.
   - Your bottom leg can be slightly bent for stability, or you can extend it out straight along the floor for an added challenge.

3. **Lift Your Leg:**

- Exhale as you lift your top leg upward towards the ceiling, keeping it straight and in line with your body.

   - Focus on using the muscles on the side of your hip to lift the leg, rather than swinging or using momentum.

4. **Controlled Lowering:**
   - Inhale as you slowly lower your leg back down to the starting position, maintaining control throughout the movement.
   - Avoid letting your leg drop suddenly or collapsing onto the mat.

5. **Repetition:**
   - Perform the desired number of repetitions on one side before switching to the other side.
   - Aim for 10-15 repetitions per side, focusing on quality of movement and maintaining proper form throughout.

Modification Options:

1. **Bent Knee Side Leg Raises:**
   - If you find straight leg raises too challenging, you can bend your top knee at a 90-degree angle and perform the raises with a bent leg.

- This modification reduces the leverage and makes the exercise easier to perform while still targeting the outer thigh and hip muscles.

2. **Wall Side Leg Raises:**
   - Perform side leg raises while standing with your side against a wall for support.
   - Place one hand on the wall for balance and stability as you lift your top leg out to the side.
   - This modification provides additional support and balance assistance, making the exercise more accessible for beginners.

Extension Exercises:

1. **Clamshells:**
   - Lie on your side with your knees bent and feet together, keeping your hips stacked and core engaged.
   - Exhale as you lift your top knee upward while keeping your feet together, opening your legs like a clamshell.
   - Inhale as you lower your knee back down with control, repeating for the desired number of repetitions.
   - This exercise targets the outer thigh and hip muscles in a slightly different range of motion.

2. **Resistance Band Side Leg Raises:**

   - Place a resistance band around your ankles or just above your knees, and perform side leg raises while lying on your side.

   - The resistance band adds extra resistance to the movement, increasing the challenge and intensity of the exercise.

Single Leg Balance

Single-leg balance exercises are excellent for improving balance, stability, and proprioception. Here are detailed instructions on how to perform single-leg balance, along with modification options and extension exercises:

1. **Starting Position:**
   - Stand tall with your feet together and your arms relaxed at your sides.
   - Shift your weight onto one foot, engaging the muscles of that leg to maintain stability.

2. **Lift Your Leg:**
   - Slowly lift the opposite foot off the ground, bending the knee and bringing it up towards your chest.
   - Keep your standing leg slightly bent to help absorb any minor adjustments in balance.

3. **Find Your Balance:**
   - Balance on the standing leg, keeping your core engaged and your gaze focused on a fixed point in front of you.
   - Aim to maintain a straight line from your head to your lifted foot, avoiding any leaning or tilting.

4. **Hold and Stabilize:**
   - Hold the position for 15-30 seconds, or longer if you feel comfortable, focusing on maintaining steady balance and control.
   - Keep your breath steady and relaxed throughout the exercise.

5. **Lower Your Leg:**
   - Slowly lower your lifted leg back down to the ground with control, returning to the starting position.
   - Take a moment to reset and stabilize before repeating the exercise on the other leg.

6. **Repeat on the Other Leg:**
   - Shift your weight onto the opposite foot and lift the other leg, following the same steps to balance on the other side.

Modification Options:

1. **Supportive Surface:**
   - Perform single-leg balance exercises near a sturdy surface, such as a wall or countertop, that you can lightly touch for support if needed.

- Lightly place your fingertips on the surface to help maintain balance while still challenging your stability.

2. **Reduce Range of Motion:**
   - If balancing on one leg is challenging, start by reducing the range of motion.
   - Instead of lifting your knee all the way up towards your chest, simply lift your foot a few inches off the ground while still keeping the knee bent.

Extension Exercises:

1. **Standing Single-Leg Balance with Arm Reach:**
   - Perform the single-leg balance exercise as described above.
   - Once you've found your balance, extend your arms out to the sides or overhead, reaching towards the ceiling.
   - This variation adds an additional challenge by incorporating upper body movement while maintaining balance on one leg.

2. **Single-Leg Balance on Unstable Surface:**
   - Stand on a foam pad, balance disc, or other unstable surface to increase the difficulty of the exercise.

- The unstable surface challenges your balance and proprioception, forcing your muscles to work harder to maintain stability.

Single Leg Romanian Deadlifts

Single-leg Romanian deadlifts are a great exercise for strengthening the hamstrings, glutes, and lower back while also improving balance and stability. Here are detailed instructions on how to perform single-leg Romanian deadlifts, along with modification options and extension exercises:

1. **Starting Position:**
   - Stand tall with your feet hip-width apart and your arms relaxed at your sides.
   - Shift your weight onto one foot and slightly bend that knee to prepare for the movement.

2. **Hinge at the Hips:**
   - Keeping your back straight and core engaged, slowly hinge forward at the hips.
   - Simultaneously, lift your non-weight-bearing leg straight back behind you, maintaining a slight bend in the standing knee.

3. **Lowering Phase:**

   - Continue hinging forward until your torso and non-weight-bearing leg are parallel to the ground, forming a straight line from head to heel.
   - Allow a natural bend in the standing knee while maintaining stability through the ankle and hip.

4. **Engage the Hamstrings:**
   - Focus on feeling a stretch in the hamstring of your standing leg as you lower your torso towards the ground.
   - Keep your hips square and avoid rotating your pelvis as you perform the movement.

5. **Return to Starting Position:**
   - Engage your hamstring and glute muscles to slowly reverse the movement, lifting your torso back up to the starting position.
   - Simultaneously, lower your non-weight-bearing leg back down towards the ground with control.

6. **Complete the Repetition:**
   - Complete the desired number of repetitions on one leg before switching to the other leg.
   - Aim for 8-12 repetitions per leg, focusing on controlled movement and maintaining proper form throughout.

Modification Options:

1. **Assisted Single-Leg Deadlifts:**
   - Perform single-leg deadlifts with the assistance of a stable surface, such as a wall or countertop.
   - Lightly touch the surface with one hand for balance and stability as you hinge forward into the movement.

2. **Partial Range of Motion:**
   - If you're new to single-leg deadlifts or have limited flexibility, reduce the range of motion.
   - Only lower your torso and non-weight-bearing leg to a comfortable level where you can maintain balance and stability without compromising form.

Extension Exercises:

1. **Single-Leg Deadlift with Dumbbells:**
   - Hold a dumbbell or kettlebell in one hand while performing the single-leg deadlift.
   - Hold the weight in the hand opposite the standing leg to add resistance and increase the challenge of the exercise.

2. **Single-Leg Deadlift with Row:**

   - Perform a single-leg deadlift with a dumbbell or kettlebell in one hand as described above.

   - At the bottom of the movement, perform a row by pulling the weight towards your hip while keeping your elbow close to your body.

   - Lower the weight back down as you return to the starting position, completing both the deadlift and row in one fluid motion.

Skater Jumps

Skater jumps are a dynamic plyometric exercise that targets multiple muscle groups, including the glutes, quadriceps, hamstrings, and calves, while also improving balance and coordination. Here are detailed instructions on how to perform skater jumps, along with modification options and extension exercises:

1. **Starting Position:**
   - Stand upright with your feet shoulder-width apart and arms relaxed at your sides.
   - Engage your core muscles to stabilize your spine and maintain proper posture throughout the exercise.

2. **Jumping Motion:**
   - Bend your knees slightly and push off explosively with your right foot, jumping laterally to the left.
   - Swing your arms to help propel your body sideways, maintaining balance and control as you jump.

3. **Mid-Air Transition:**
   - Land softly on your left foot, bending the knee to absorb the impact of the landing.

- Allow your right foot to swing behind your left leg, mimicking the motion of a speed skater.

4. **Continuous Movement:**
   - Immediately push off with your left foot and jump laterally to the right, swinging your arms and transitioning smoothly between jumps.
   - Land softly on your right foot, bending the knee to absorb the impact, and allow your left foot to swing behind your right leg.

5. **Repeat the Sequence:**
   - Continue jumping laterally from side to side, mimicking the motion of a speed skater gliding across the ice.
   - Aim for a fluid and rhythmic motion, maintaining balance and control throughout the exercise.

6. **Repetition:**
   - Perform the skater jumps for the desired number of repetitions or time, focusing on explosive power and proper form.

Modification Options:

1. **Reduce Intensity:**
   - If you're new to skater jumps or have limited mobility, you can perform a modified version by reducing the intensity of the movement.
   - Instead of jumping laterally, step sideways from one foot to the other, focusing on controlled movement and balance.

2. **Use Support:**
   - Perform skater jumps near a sturdy surface, such as a wall or countertop, that you can lightly touch for support if needed.
   - Lightly place your fingertips on the surface to help maintain balance and stability while still challenging yourself with the exercise.

Extension Exercises:

1. **Skater Jumps with Touch:**
   - Perform skater jumps as described above, but add a touch to the ground with your fingertips each time you land on one foot.
   - This variation increases the range of motion and adds an additional challenge to the exercise.

2. **Skater Jumps with Cross:**

   - Perform skater jumps as described above, but add a cross-body arm movement with each jump.

   - As you jump laterally to the left, swing your right arm across your body towards your left foot, and vice versa.

   - This variation engages the core muscles more intensely and improves coordination.

Speed Skaters

Speed skaters are a dynamic plyometric exercise that targets multiple muscle groups, including the glutes, quadriceps, hamstrings, and calves, while also improving cardiovascular fitness and agility. Here are detailed instructions on how to perform speed skaters, along with modification options and extension exercises:

1. **Starting Position:**
   - Stand upright with your feet hip-width apart and your arms relaxed at your sides.
   - Engage your core muscles to stabilize your spine and maintain proper posture throughout the exercise.

2. **Jumping Motion:**
   - Bend your knees slightly and push off explosively with your right foot, jumping diagonally to the left.
   - Swing your right arm across your body towards your left foot, and allow your left arm to swing behind you for balance.

3. **Mid-Air Transition:**
   - Land softly on your left foot, bending the knee to absorb the impact of the landing.

- Simultaneously, swing your left arm across your body towards your right foot, and allow your right arm to swing behind you.

4. **Continuous Movement:**
   - Immediately push off with your left foot and jump diagonally to the right, swinging your arms and transitioning smoothly between jumps.
   - Land softly on your right foot, bending the knee to absorb the impact, and repeat the jumping motion to the opposite side.

5. **Repeat the Sequence:**
   - Continue jumping diagonally from side to side, mimicking the motion of a speed skater gliding across the ice.
   - Aim for a fluid and rhythmic motion, maintaining balance and control throughout the exercise.

6. **Repetition:**
   - Perform the speed skaters for the desired number of repetitions or time, focusing on explosive power and proper form.

Modification Options:

1. **Reduce Intensity:**
   - If you're new to speed skaters or have limited mobility, you can perform a modified version by reducing the intensity of the movement.
   - Instead of jumping explosively, step diagonally from one foot to the other, focusing on controlled movement and balance.

2. **Use Support:**
   - Perform speed skaters near a sturdy surface, such as a wall or countertop, that you can lightly touch for support if needed.
   - Lightly place your fingertips on the surface to help maintain balance and stability while still challenging yourself with the exercise.

Extension Exercises:

1. **Speed Skaters with Hop:**
   - Perform speed skaters as described above, but add a small hop with each jump to increase the intensity of the exercise.

   - Focus on exploding off the ground with each jump and landing softly to absorb the impact.

2. **Speed Skaters with Cross-Body Reach:**
   - Perform speed skaters as described above, but add a cross-body arm movement with each jump.
   - As you jump diagonally to the left, swing your right arm across your body towards your left foot, and vice versa.
   - This variation engages the core muscles more intensely and improves coordination.

Squats

Bodyweight squats are a fundamental lower body exercise that targets the quadriceps, hamstrings, glutes, and core muscles. Here are detailed instructions on how to perform bodyweight squats, along with modification options and extension exercises:

1. **Starting Position:**
   - Stand with your feet slightly wider than shoulder-width apart, toes pointed slightly outward.
   - Keep your chest lifted, shoulders back, and core engaged throughout the exercise.

2. **Lowering Phase:**
   - Inhale as you bend your knees and hips, lowering your body down into a squat position.
   - Keep your weight in your heels, and lower your hips back and down as if you were sitting back into a chair.

3. **Squat Depth:**
   - Descend until your thighs are parallel to the ground or as low as comfortable while maintaining proper form.

- Ensure your knees stay aligned with your toes and do not collapse inward.

4. **Pressing Phase:**
   - Exhale as you push through your heels to straighten your legs and return to the starting position.
   - Squeeze your glutes at the top of the movement to fully engage the muscles.

5. **Repetition:**
   - Perform the desired number of repetitions, focusing on controlled movement and maintaining proper form throughout.

Modification Options:

1. **Chair Squats:**
   - Perform squats by lowering yourself onto a chair or bench, lightly tapping the surface before standing back up.
   - This modification reduces the depth of the squat and can be helpful for those with limited mobility or strength.

2. **Half Squats:**

- Perform squats to a shallower depth, stopping when your thighs are halfway between standing and a full squat position.
    - This modification reduces the range of motion and can be useful for beginners or those working on form.

Extension Exercises:

1. **Jump Squats:**
    - Perform a regular bodyweight squat, but explode off the ground as you rise up, jumping into the air.
    - Land softly and immediately lower back down into the squat position to complete one repetition.

2. **Squat Jumps:**
    - Start in a squat position and explosively jump as high as you can, reaching your arms overhead.
    - Land softly with bent knees and immediately lower back down into the squat position to complete one repetition.

3. **Squat Pulses:**
    - Perform a regular squat, but instead of returning to the starting position, pulse up and down in a small range of motion.

- Maintain tension in the muscles throughout the pulsing motion to increase time under tension.

4. **Squat to Calf Raises:**
   - Perform a regular squat, but as you rise up, come onto the balls of your feet to perform a calf raise.
   - Lower back down into the squat position and repeat the movement, alternating between squats and calf raises.

5. **Sumo Squats:**
   - Stand with your feet wider than shoulder-width apart and toes pointed outward.
   - Perform squats in this wide stance, targeting the inner thighs and glutes.

6. **Sumo Squats with Calf Raises:**
   - Perform sumo squats as described above, but add a calf raise at the top of each squat.
   - This variation targets both the inner thighs and calves for a comprehensive lower body workout.

7. **Squat Jacks:**
   - Start in a squat position with your feet together and knees bent.

- Jump explosively into the air while simultaneously spreading your legs wide and bringing your arms overhead.

- Land softly in a wide squat position, then immediately jump back to the starting position with your feet together.

- Repeat the movement for the desired number of repetitions, focusing on speed and agility.

8. **Side-Leg Squats:**

- Stand with your feet wider than shoulder-width apart and toes pointed slightly outward.

- Lower your body down into a squat position, then shift your weight to one side and lift the opposite leg out to the side.

- Return to the squat position and repeat on the other side, alternating sides with each repetition.

- This variation targets the inner and outer thighs, as well as the glutes, providing a different challenge compared to traditional squats.

Standing Quad Stretch

Incorporate the standing quad stretch and its variations into your warm-up or cool-down routine to improve flexibility and mobility in the quadriceps and hip flexors. Here are detailed instructions on how to perform standing quad stretches, along with modification options and extension exercises:

1. **Starting Position:**
   - Stand tall with your feet together and your arms relaxed at your sides.

2. **Shift Your Weight:**
   - Shift your weight onto one leg while keeping the other foot flat on the ground.

3. **Bend Your Knee:**
   - Bend the knee of the leg that you're not standing on, bringing your heel towards your buttocks.

4. **Grasp Your Foot:**
   - Reach back with the hand on the same side as the bent leg and grasp your ankle or foot.

5. **Maintain Balance:**
   - Keep your knees close together and your thighs aligned vertically to maximize the stretch.
   - Engage your core muscles to stabilize your spine and maintain proper posture throughout the stretch.

6. **Hold the Stretch:**
   - Hold the stretch for 20-30 seconds, feeling the stretch along the front of the thigh and hip of the bent leg.
   - Focus on breathing deeply and evenly to help relax into the stretch.

7. **Release and Switch Sides:**
   - Gently release your foot and return to the starting position.
   - Repeat the stretch on the opposite leg by shifting your weight onto the other leg and repeating the steps.

Modification Options:

1. **Wall Support:**
   - Perform the standing quad stretch next to a wall or sturdy object that you can lightly touch for support if needed.

- Lightly rest your hand against the wall to help maintain balance while performing the stretch.

2. **Chair Support:**
   - Perform the standing quad stretch while holding onto the back of a chair or countertop for added stability.
   - This modification is helpful for individuals who may have difficulty balancing on one leg.

Extension Exercises:

1. **Dynamic Quad Stretch:**
   - Perform the standing quad stretch as described above, but instead of holding the stretch statically, gently rock back and forth to increase mobility and flexibility in the quadriceps.

2. **Pigeon Pose:**
   - Start in a standing position and step one foot back, crossing it behind the other leg.
   - Bend your front knee and lower down into a lunge position, keeping your back leg straight.
   - Sink your hips down towards the ground and lean forward, feeling a deep stretch in the front of the hip and thigh of the back leg.

- Hold the stretch for 20-30 seconds, then switch sides to stretch the opposite hip and thigh.

Standing Side Bends

Incorporate standing side bends and their variations into your core workout routine to strengthen and tone the oblique muscles, improve lateral flexibility, and enhance overall posture. Here are detailed instructions on how to perform side bends, along with modification options and extension exercises:

1. **Starting Position:**
   - Stand tall with your feet hip-width apart and your arms relaxed at your sides.

2. **Engage Your Core:**
   - Engage your abdominal muscles by drawing your belly button towards your spine to stabilize your torso.

3. **Lower to One Side:**
   - Slowly lower your torso to one side, keeping your spine straight and your shoulders level.
   - Imagine sliding your hand down the side of your thigh as you bend, reaching towards your knee or shin.

4. **Stretch and Hold:**

- Feel the stretch along the side of your torso and waist on the opposite side.
   - Hold the stretch for 20-30 seconds, breathing deeply and maintaining a steady rhythm.

5. **Return to Center:**
   - Slowly return to the upright position, engaging your core muscles to lift your torso back to the center.
   - Keep your movements controlled and avoid leaning forward or backward.

6. **Repeat on the Other Side:**
   - Lower your torso to the opposite side, feeling the stretch along the opposite side of your torso.
   - Hold the stretch for 20-30 seconds before returning to the center.

7. **Alternate Sides:**
   - Repeat the side bends for several repetitions on each side, focusing on smooth and controlled movement.

Modification Options:

1. **Reduced Range of Motion:**

- If you have limited flexibility or mobility, you can perform smaller side bends with a reduced range of motion.
   - Focus on engaging the core muscles and maintaining proper alignment while bending to the side.

2. **Chair Support:**
   - Perform the standing side bends while holding onto the back of a chair or countertop for added stability.
   - This modification can help you maintain balance and focus on proper form while performing the exercise.

Extension Exercises:

1. **Weighted Side Bends:**
   - Hold a dumbbell or kettlebell in one hand while performing the standing side bends to add resistance to the exercise.
   - Keep your movements slow and controlled, focusing on engaging the oblique muscles to lift the weight.

2. **Standing Side Crunches:**
   - Start in the standing position with your hands behind your head and elbows pointing out to the sides.

- Perform a side bend to one side while simultaneously lifting the knee on the same side towards the elbow.

- Focus on contracting the oblique muscles as you bend to the side, feeling the crunch along the side of your torso.

- Return to the starting position and repeat on the other side.

Supermans

Incorporate Supermans and their variations into your back strengthening routine to target the erector spinae muscles, improve spinal stability, and reduce the risk of lower back pain. Here are detailed instructions on how to perform supermans, along with modification options and extension exercises:

1. **Starting Position:**
   - Lie face down on a mat or the floor with your arms extended overhead and your legs straight.
   - Keep your neck in a neutral position by looking down towards the ground.

2. **Engage Your Core:**
   - Engage your abdominal muscles to stabilize your spine and support your lower back throughout the exercise.

3. **Lift Upper Body and Legs:**
   - Simultaneously lift your chest, arms, and legs off the ground by contracting your lower back muscles.
   - Keep your arms and legs straight as you lift, aiming to create a "flying" position with your body.

4. **Squeeze Your Glutes:**
   - Squeeze your glutes at the top of the movement to further engage your lower back muscles.
   - Focus on lifting your chest and thighs as high as comfortably possible while maintaining control.

5. **Hold and Squeeze:**
   - Hold the top position for a few seconds, focusing on squeezing your lower back muscles to maintain the lift.
   - Keep your neck relaxed and avoid straining or arching your back excessively.

6. **Lower Back Down:**
   - Slowly lower your chest, arms, and legs back down to the starting position, maintaining control and resisting the urge to collapse.
   - Allow your muscles to relax briefly before performing the next repetition.

7. **Repeat the Movement:**
   - Perform the Supermans for the desired number of repetitions, focusing on quality over quantity.

- Keep your movements controlled and maintain proper form throughout the exercise.

Modification Options:

1. **Alternating Arm and Leg Lifts:**
   - If lifting both arms and legs simultaneously is too challenging, you can perform alternating arm and leg lifts.
   - Lift one arm and the opposite leg off the ground at the same time, then switch sides and repeat.

2. **Reduced Range of Motion:**
   - If you have limited flexibility or mobility, you can reduce the range of motion by lifting your chest, arms, and legs only a few inches off the ground.
   - Focus on engaging the lower back muscles and maintaining proper alignment while performing the exercise.

Extension Exercises:

1. **Superman Pulses:**
   - Perform the Supermans as described above, but instead of holding the top position, pulse up and down in a small range of motion.

- Focus on contracting and squeezing your lower back muscles with each pulse, increasing the intensity of the exercise.

2. **Weighted Supermans:**
   - Hold a light dumbbell or resistance band in your hands while performing the Supermans to add resistance to the exercise.
   - Keep your movements slow and controlled, focusing on engaging the lower back muscles to lift the weight.

Tricep Dips

Incorporate tricep dips and their variations into your upper body workout routine to strengthen and tone the tricep muscles, improve arm strength, and enhance overall upper body definition. Here are detailed instructions on how to perform tricep dips, along with modification options and extension exercises:

1. **Starting Position:**
   - Sit on the edge of a sturdy chair, bench, or elevated surface with your hands placed shoulder-width apart beside your hips.
   - Grip the edge of the chair firmly with your fingers pointing towards your body.
   - Extend your legs in front of you with your heels planted on the floor, knees bent at a 90-degree angle.

2. **Engage Your Core:**
   - Engage your abdominal muscles to stabilize your torso and maintain proper posture throughout the exercise.

3. **Lower Your Body:**

- Press into your hands to lift your hips off the chair and slide forward slightly, keeping your back close to the edge of the chair.
   - Lower your body by bending your elbows, allowing them to flare out to the sides.
   - Lower yourself until your elbows are bent at approximately 90 degrees, or until your upper arms are parallel to the ground.

4. **Push Back Up:**
   - Press through your palms to straighten your arms and lift your body back up to the starting position.
   - Keep your shoulders down and away from your ears as you push back up.

5. **Repeat the Movement:**
   - Perform the tricep dips for the desired number of repetitions, focusing on maintaining proper form and control throughout the exercise.
   - Keep your movements slow and controlled, avoiding any jerky or swinging motions.

Modification Options:

1. **Tricep Dips on Chair:**
   - Perform the tricep dips on a sturdy chair or bench with your legs extended in front of you and your feet flat on the floor.
   - Keep your hands shoulder-width apart on the edge of the chair and follow the same movement pattern as described above.

2. **Bent-Knee Tricep Dips:**
   - If performing the tricep dips with straight legs is too challenging, you can bend your knees and place your feet flat on the floor for added stability.
   - Follow the same movement pattern as described above, focusing on engaging the tricep muscles as you lower and lift your body.

Extension Exercises:

1. **Tricep Dips with Leg Extension:**
   - Perform the tricep dips as described above, but as you push back up to the starting position, extend one leg straight out in front of you.
   - Hold the extended leg parallel to the ground for a few seconds before returning it to the starting position.

- Repeat the movement with the opposite leg, alternating legs with each repetition.

2. **Weighted Tricep Dips:**
   - Hold a dumbbell or weighted object on your lap while performing the tricep dips to add resistance to the exercise.
   - Increase the weight gradually as you build strength and endurance in the tricep muscles.

Tricep Kickbacks

Incorporate tricep kickbacks and their variations into your upper body workout routine to strengthen and tone the tricep muscles, improve arm definition, and enhance overall upper body strength. Here are detailed instructions on how to perform tricep kickbacks, along with modification options and extension exercises:

1. **Starting Position:**
   - Stand with your feet hip-width apart and hold a dumbbell in each hand.
   - Hinge forward at the hips to bring your torso parallel to the ground, keeping your back straight and core engaged.
   - Bend your elbows to a 90-degree angle, with your upper arms parallel to the ground and your palms facing each other.

2. **Extend Your Arms:**
   - Keeping your upper arms stationary, straighten your elbows and extend your arms back behind you.
   - Focus on contracting your tricep muscles as you fully extend your arms, squeezing them at the top of the movement.

3. **Hold and Squeeze:**

   - Hold the fully extended position for a brief moment, feeling the contraction in your triceps.

   - Keep your wrists firm and your shoulders down, avoiding any swinging or momentum.

4. **Return to Starting Position:**

   - Slowly bend your elbows to return to the starting position, maintaining control throughout the movement.

   - Keep your upper arms parallel to the ground and avoid swinging the weights.

5. **Repeat the Movement:**

   - Perform the tricep kickbacks for the desired number of repetitions, focusing on smooth and controlled movements.

   - Keep your core engaged and your back straight throughout the exercise to stabilize your body.

Modification Options:

1. **Lighter Weights:**

- If you're new to tricep kickbacks or find them challenging, start with lighter weights to ensure proper form and technique.
  - Gradually increase the weight as you become more comfortable with the exercise and build strength in your triceps.

2. **One-Arm Kickbacks:**
  - Perform the tricep kickbacks one arm at a time if using both arms simultaneously is too difficult.
  - Focus on maintaining stability in your torso and minimizing rotation as you extend and lower each arm individually.

Extension Exercises:

1. **Overhead Tricep Extension:**
  - Stand with your feet hip-width apart and hold a dumbbell or kettlebell with both hands overhead.
  - Lower the weight behind your head by bending your elbows, keeping your upper arms close to your ears.
  - Extend your arms fully to raise the weight back overhead, focusing on contracting your tricep muscles.

- Repeat for the desired number of repetitions, maintaining control throughout the movement.

2. **Tricep Pushdowns:**
   - Attach a resistance band or cable machine to a high anchor point.
   - Stand facing the anchor point with your feet hip-width apart and grab the handles with an overhand grip.
   - Keep your elbows close to your sides as you push the handles down towards the ground, fully extending your arms.
   - Return to the starting position with control, focusing on the contraction in your triceps.
   - Repeat for the desired number of repetitions, keeping your core engaged and your back straight.

V-ups

Incorporate V-ups and their variations into your core workout routine to strengthen and tone the abdominal muscles, improve core stability, and enhance overall posture. Here are detailed instructions on how to perform v-ups, along with modification options and extension exercises:

1. **Starting Position:**
   - Lie flat on your back with your arms extended overhead and your legs straight.
   - Engage your core muscles by drawing your belly button towards your spine to stabilize your torso.

2. **Lift Upper Body and Legs:**
   - Simultaneously lift your upper body and legs off the ground, keeping them straight.
   - Reach your arms towards your feet as you lift, aiming to touch your toes or shins.

3. **Form a V Shape:**
   - Continue lifting until your body forms a "V" shape, balancing on your tailbone.

  - Keep your legs straight and your toes pointed towards the ceiling throughout the movement.

4. **Contract Your Abs:**
  - Squeeze your abdominal muscles at the top of the movement, focusing on the contraction.
  - Maintain control and avoid using momentum to swing your body.

5. **Lower Back Down:**
  - Slowly lower your upper body and legs back down to the starting position, maintaining tension in your core muscles.
  - Avoid letting your shoulders or feet touch the ground between repetitions.

6. **Repeat the Movement:**
  - Perform the V-ups for the desired number of repetitions, focusing on quality over quantity.
  - Keep your movements controlled and maintain proper form throughout the exercise.

Modification Options:

1. **Bent-Knee V-Ups:**

- If you find it challenging to keep your legs straight, you can perform the V-ups with your knees bent.

- Lift your upper body and legs towards each other, aiming to touch your knees instead of your toes.

2. **Leg Raises:**

- Lie flat on your back with your arms at your sides and your legs straight.

- Lift your legs towards the ceiling, keeping them straight and together, until they are perpendicular to the floor.

- Lower your legs back down to the starting position without letting them touch the ground.

Extension Exercises:

1. **Weighted V-Ups:**

- Hold a dumbbell or medicine ball in your hands while performing the V-ups to add resistance to the exercise.

- This added weight increases the intensity of the exercise and helps build strength in the abdominal muscles.

2. **Alternating V-Ups:**

- Perform the V-ups as described above, but alternate reaching towards one foot at a time instead of reaching towards both feet simultaneously.
- This variation adds a rotational component to the exercise, engaging the oblique muscles as well as the rectus abdominis.

Experiment with different modification options and extension exercises to tailor the exercise to your individual needs and goals, gradually progressing towards greater core strength and definition.

Wall Sits

Incorporate wall sits and their variations into your lower body workout routine to strengthen the quadriceps, glutes, and core muscles. Here are detailed instructions on how to perform wall sits, along with modification options and extension exercises:

1. **Starting Position:**
   - Stand with your back against a wall and your feet shoulder-width apart.
   - Lower your body down until your thighs are parallel to the floor, forming a 90-degree angle at your knees.
   - Keep your back pressed against the wall and your hands resting on your thighs or at your sides for balance.

2. **Engage Your Muscles:**
   - Engage your core muscles to stabilize your spine and maintain proper posture throughout the exercise.
   - Press your lower back against the wall to prevent arching.

3. **Hold the Position:**

- Hold the wall sit position for the desired amount of time, aiming for 30 seconds to 1 minute or longer if you can.
  - Focus on breathing deeply and evenly to help maintain endurance.

4. **Repetition:**
  - Repeat the wall sit for multiple sets with adequate rest in between, gradually increasing the duration or number of sets as you progress.

Modification Options:

1. **Shallower Wall Sit:**
  - If holding a full wall sit is too challenging, start by lowering down to a shallower angle, such as a 45-degree bend at the knees.
  - Gradually increase the depth of the wall sit as you build strength and endurance.

2. **Assisted Wall Sit:**
  - Place a stability ball between your back and the wall to provide support and assistance during the wall sit.

- This modification can help reduce the intensity of the exercise while still allowing you to work on proper form and technique.

Extension Exercises:

1. **Wall Sit with Leg Lifts:**
   - Perform a wall sit as described above, maintaining the position with your thighs parallel to the floor.
   - While holding the wall sit, lift one leg off the ground and extend it straight out in front of you.
   - Hold the leg lift for a few seconds before returning the foot to the floor and repeating on the other side.
   - Alternate leg lifts for the desired number of repetitions, focusing on stability and control.

2. **Wall Sit with Ball Squeeze:**
   - Place a small exercise ball or cushion between your knees while performing the wall sit.
   - Squeeze the ball with your thighs to engage the inner thigh muscles while holding the wall sit position.
   - Hold the squeeze for a few seconds before releasing and repeating for the desired number of repetitions.

www.ingramcontent.com/pod-product-compliance
Lightning Source LLC
Chambersburg PA
CBHW051552250726
48653CB00004BA/1105